MYSTERY IN WESTERN MEDICINE

Mystery in Western Medicine

DAVID GREAVES
Centre for Philosophy and Health Care
University of Wales, Swansea

Avebury

Aldershot · Brookfield USA · Hong Kong · Singapore · Sydney

Published by
Avebury
Ashgate Publishing Ltd
Gower House
Croft Road
Aldershot
Hants GU11 3HR
England

Ashgate Publishing Company
Old Post Road
Brookfield
Vermont 05036
USA

British Library Cataloguing in Publication Data

Greaves, David
    Mystery in Western medicine. - (Avebury series in
    philosophy)
    1. Medicine - Philosophy
    I. Title
    610.1

    ISBN 1 85972 441 8

Library of Congress Catalog Card Number: 96-85196

Printed in Great Britain by the Ipswich Book Company, Suffolk

Contents

Acknowledgements

T his book has had a long gestation. It began when I was working in the Department of Epidemiology and Preventive Medicine (now the Department of Public Health) at Glasgow University. There I began to consider the question of the status of disease and of disease classifications, and first expressed these thoughts in a presentation to a departmental seminar in 1974, which was entitled 'Classifications are Merely Useful'. In 1976 I had the opportunity to develop these ideas further when I spent a year at the MRC Medical Sociology Unit, at that time based in Aberdeen. After working in the health service for some years I joined the Centre of Medical Law and Ethics at King's College London, and again returned to a consideration of concepts of health, illness and disease. At each of these institutions I had the chance to meet and discuss my ideas with students and colleagues, and I owe a great deal to them. Without the wide range of experience and different perspectives which they have given me I could not have begun to formulate this thesis.

This then was the background, and the actual work of preparing and writing the book began in 1990 after I had joined the Centre for Philosophy and Health Care at Swansea. I have discussed several of the chapters with my colleagues at Centre seminars, and am grateful to all of them for the help and support they have given me. I would also like to thank Tina Posner, who took the time to discuss her work on diabetes with me.

Two of my colleagues deserve special mention. First, Richard Bryden whose scholarly and meticulous approach has proved invaluable. His breadth of reading and clear understanding of so many fields have been incomparable assets in directing my efforts. I cannot praise his help and advice too highly. Second, Martyn Evans undertook to read and comment on the whole book whilst in draft form, and his observations have also been of great help.

Finally, because I have not yet succumbed to pressures to use a word processor, Gwyneth Abbott has kindly typed and retyped the book during the many stages it has been through. My thanks go to her for her help and patience with this onerous task.

1 Introduction

I n the late twentieth century western medicine faces a perplexing paradox. On the one hand the system of medicine that has been developed over the past two or three hundred years has reached a stage of unprecedented technological success, but on the other hand the health care policies of those developed countries from which it has been derived, are faltering and under such severe strain as to be facing serious challenges almost everywhere. The problem for planners is presented as one of escalating costs failing to deal with ever-increasing unmet needs; and as the technological success of western medicine has gradually been followed by its spread to all parts of the world, developing countries, with low national incomes, are being affected even more acutely. Something has to change and the principal response has been to look to institutional and managerial reforms to resolve these issues.

The purpose of this study is to show that such reforms, when taken alone, are not sufficient in themselves, because they only deal with problems as they arise on the surface. What is required is a deepseated reflection which recognises and faces up to the false assumptions of the past, and is prepared to rethink questions about the nature of medicine and the goals of health care. This must then be followed by a collective change of consciousness and of attitudes throughout society.

This study then will develop the basis for a critique of western medicine aimed at providing an analysis sufficient to this task, starting from the proposition that any system of medicine must necessarily embody a mysterious quality. What is meant here by mystery is an all-encompassing element of indeterminacy, such that there is always a degree of uncertainty in both the theory and practice of medicine. The failure to recognise that this applies to modern western medicine has led to serious misunderstandings and distortions in both medical theory and practice. This failure has meant that the accepted justification for the foundation of western medicine cannot be sustained. It is also a crucial flaw in most of the recent major critiques of western medicine, limiting the insights which collectively they have been able to develop.

The claim will be made that in all cultures of which we have knowledge, both historical and contemporary, only the recent western tradition has denied the essential place of the mysterious in the understanding and explanation of health, illness, disease and the role of medicine. The recognition of a mysterious quality in medicine is almost universal and derives from the perception that medicine is not a unitary and objective system in the sense of being independent of social beliefs, values and practices. This mysterious quality is pervasive and permeates medical knowledge, including that perspective which emphasises rationality and reason. It is only in western medicine since the nineteenth century that these latter qualities have been seen to be freed from mystery to an extent that has not been known previously. It is also the basis on which the medical profession and the medical model of disease, treatment and care have been developed and are seen as being both scientifically based and effective.

The main proposition underlying the study is therefore that any system of medicine necessarily contains an inseparable meld of both mysterious and rational qualities. Hence the aim will be to show that the claim that modern western medicine derives almost exclusively from the latter is more to do with ideology and image than reality.

However, the denial of the mysterious has had serious consequences and its recognition allows for their reappraisal. The study will therefore begin with an analysis of what is meant by mystery and its relationship with medicine. This will then be considered more specifically in re-evaluating how some aspects of western medicine have been operated in theory and practice over recent centuries, and it will involve an analysis of the way that western medicine has been developed so as to produce a reinterpretation or marginalisation of all that is not quantifiable or wholly comprehensible in terms of a particular conception of rationality. It is best illustrated by considering what are seen as persistently 'problematic' or 'anomalous' elements of situations which are resistant to causal explanations, i.e. those which are regarded as either 'non-rational' or 'irrational' and yet continue to resist causal explanations despite all attempts to deal with them. Such scenarios challenge the unity of the western medical system and so provide a clue to the mysterious. They include the failure of orthodox medicine to accommodate alternative medicine on an equal footing and of certain aspects of general practice and public health to fit the traditional medical model; the inability to resolve questions of resource allocation because of the denial or exclusion both of issues of subjectivity and of the social determination of what is to count as a medical problem; the frequent lack of patient compliance with medical advice; and the persistent difficulty in developing and changing professional health care roles.

This analysis will then be used to reassess some of the best known critiques of western medicine, which in ignoring the mysterious and accepting the thesis of the uncomplicated way in which rationalism has determined the course of modern western medicine, have made assumptions about the way in which it operates. This has left two key and interlocking elements unquestioned. First, that medicine has been shaped by and is dependent on a positivist conception of science, and second that the medical profession has relied on paternalism and beneficence in establishing its authority and power. The role of these two elements is central to many critiques, because they have been conceived in relation to them. Therefore, to take issue with the role attributed to them strikes at both the fundamental claims of western medicine and the basis of the criticisms and remedies offered by the critiques.

The insights gained from this analysis and re-evaluation will then be used to develop the outline of a different approach which will indicate ways in which western medicine should be modified in both theory and practice. This will begin with the recognition that although the present justification of western medicine is flawed, a more adequate one may be found through re-examining current medical practice and re-orientating it by taking account of particular themes in other contemporary and historical systems of medicine. The unrecognised thread which unites and gives coherence to all these medical systems is the role of mystery. It must be wholeheartedly acknowledged if the current mistakes and problems of western medicine are to be revealed and understood, so that more plausible moral and scientific foundations of western medicine can be established.

2 Medicine and mystery

A central tenet in our understanding of the role of western medicine is that it involves a programme of inevitable progress, because the goal being pursued is unified and objective. This is further allied to the view that it is only through scientific rationalism that such a process is possible. Taken together this complex of beliefs, relating to both theory and practice may be referred to as a positivist conception of science (or scientific positivism, sometimes abbreviated to scientism). This runs in parallel with the wider tradition of western thought which has been represented as follows:

> ... from Plato to our own day, the overwhelming majority of systematic thinkers of all schools, whether rationalists, idealists, phenomenalists, positivists or empiricists have, despite their many radical differences, proceeded on one central assumption: that reality, whatever appearances may indicate, is in essence a rational whole where all things ultimately cohere. They suppose that there exists (at least in principle) a body of discoverable truths touching all conceivable questions, both theoretical and practical; that there is, and can be, only one correct method or set of methods for gaining access to these truths; and that these truths, as well as the methods used in their discovery, are universally valid.(1)

Western medicine is not then unique in being influenced by this central assumption but it has been affected by it in a particular manner, through which the notion of mystery has been excluded.

This chapter will therefore explore various different ways in which the role of mystery might be interpreted in relation to medicine, once the central assumption outlined above has been seen as open to challenge. The purpose of this will be to identify a number of strands in developing an account of the mysterious in western medicine, through which to analyse different facets of it and which it is not usually possible to scrutinise.

One definition of mystery given in the *Oxford English Dictionary* is 'hidden or inexplicable matter'(2) and it is this which will be used as a focus, being considered to begin with in relation to two particular medical notions. The first could be described as involving a puzzle to which it is believed that the solution is available though it has not yet been revealed. Imagine a case of a patient who has chronic bronchitis with frequent bouts of breathlessness during which he coughs up sputum. He has regular medication which he takes when these episodes begin, and they usually get better within a few days. However, one particular attack does not respond to treatment and after a week there has been no improvement in his condition. This is a new experience for the patient, such that he may say that it is a mystery to him as to why he should not have improved. He therefore decides to seek advice from his general practitioner, who after taking a history and examining the patient, makes a diagnosis of pneumonia and changes the medication accordingly, at the same time advising the patient to stay at home. Three days later the condition of the patient has worsened, and the general practitioner is puzzled as to why there should have been this lack of response. He may then say to the patient that it is a mystery to him, and the best hope for discovering the truth about it is for the patient to go to hospital for further investigations. These then reveal that the patient does not have pneumonia, and the hospital doctor considers he might have an unusual heart condition, although the range of tests available neither confirms nor excludes this diagnosis with certainty. Nevertheless treatment is started for this condition, but unfortunately it is without benefit and shortly afterwards the patient dies. The hospital doctor might also then say that he is mystified as to the condition which the patient was suffering from and why he should have died from it. Hence his response is to ask the relatives for their agreement to a pathologist carrying out a post-mortem examination in order to establish a diagnosis for the condition which caused the death. This then reveals that although there were some pathological changes in both the lungs and the heart, there is not a clearcut disease process in either to which death may be readily attributed. However, the law requires that a sufficient cause be given on the death certificate, so that the pathologist despite regarding the death as something of a mystery will be constrained to state a case in terms of disease conditions, although he can do no more than make a best guess as to what they might be.

What emerges from this case history is that reference has been made to the mysterious nature of the patient's condition at every stage, first by the patient, then the general practitioner, the hospital doctor and the pathologist. However, in each instance this mysteriousness, which can be described in terms of hidden matter, is not thought to be ultimately impenetrable, but only so in relation to the knowledge and expertise of the relevant participant at that stage. What this reflects is a hierarchy, such that matter which is hidden at a lower level will be expected to be revealed for what it truly is and thereby made explicable at a higher level, and this revelation of true knowledge can be expected to emerge at any successive level.

6

So if for example, the general practitioner said to the patient 'your condition is a mystery to me', he would mean precisely that it was a mystery *to him*, but not that he thought it a mystery beyond resolution. This then applies equally at each stage, as the use of the word mystery in this context refers to hidden matter which presents a puzzle not yet solved, but which it is believed can be unravelled through the application of knowledge and expertise already available at a superior level. So what is being referred to is a hidden quality which has the possibility of being revealed, and this contrasts with an inevitably indeterminate quality where the mystery can never be explained.

A further problem arises though, because if each successive level of expertise fails to solve the puzzle the pathologist is seen to be the final arbiter, and yet, as in the case described, he may also be unable to resolve the mystery. In this event it would seem that we do have a 'real' mystery, that is hidden matter which western medicine has failed to reduce to a soluble puzzle. But no such acknowledgement is made, and a second line of reasoning is introduced to deal with this situation. This recognises that western medicine does not yet have the complete answer to all such puzzles, but confidently believes that it will have the means to solve them eventually. The ability of the pathologist to make a best guess in writing the death certificate rests on this belief, and is in effect a statement that he has already partially solved the puzzle which further knowledge would enable him to refine in future, so making his best guess completely accurate.

Contrary to this it might appear that the pathologist could accept the possibility of his being mistaken, or even admit that we cannot know with certainty that our knowledge is completely accurate. However the system within which he works does not allow for this, and takes for granted that the resolution of medical uncertainty follows because potentially all aspects of medical knowledge are open to inspection. So, for example, the currently accepted classifications of disease list a number of medical conditions for which there are one or more recognised causes, but where in addition there are some cases where the cause is unknown. The cause is then described as idiopathic, indicating that all possible known causes must be considered in each case, but where this search proves unsuccessful it must be admitted that there is no presently recognised explanation for the condition. The label idiopathic is therefore a diagnosis by exclusion, but importantly it also denotes an expectation that in future medical science will, or at least has the potential to, find a cause for each case. In other words it represents a belief in the ability of medical science to resolve the present mystery.

A further aspect of this follows from the way in which medical science is seen as dealing with idiopathic conditions. The assumption is made that cases of a particular condition referred to as idiopathic will eventually be revealed to be part of either one or a number of discrete disease entities. An example is that of cot (or crib) deaths, which occur suddenly and unexpectedly in the first few months of life and for which there is no accepted medical cause. Despite this it was stated at an International Conference in 1969 that 'Sudden Infant Death Syndrome (SIDS) is a real disease, not a vague mysterious killer'(3) and later that the word syndrome 'had the important virtue of communicating to the medical profession the concept that this is, in fact, a distinct clinico-pathological entity(4). So although no cause has been established for the cot deaths the claim is being made that this is a disease entity, implying that there must be a cause of a particular kind which can be discovered and through which the mystery can potentially be resolved. The use of the word syndrome is an important link in this chain of thought because it provides what are seen as legitimate grounds for the belief that there must be a cause and hence a real disease. The term syndrome is therefore being used as both a staging post in establishing the presence of a new disease, and as an indicator of faith in the scientific character of medical practice. Pronouncing that cot deaths result from the Sudden Infant Death Syndrome is to herald a new disease or diseases and simultaneously to proclaim that medical science expects to find their cause and cure given time. So these two aspects of medical mystery, its definition and its resolution are inextricably bound together and hence jointly dealt with. Once again the notion of mystery which this refers to is of something hidden rather than of something impenetrable.

For western medicine this notion of mystery as hidden matter is only of a contingent mystery, the meaning of the word being thereby redefined as merely lack of knowledge and expertise which is either already available or will be so in future. In this interpretation the word mystery seems misplaced, because the hidden matter is only so in a very limited sense. As already indicated a more appropriate description might be to refer not to medical mysteries but to medical puzzles, and to see western medicine as first converting what were once mysteries into puzzles, and then through research solving each of these puzzles in turn. What is then clear is that the sense of mystery is dispelled even if the substituted puzzle has not been and may not be solved. Terms such as idiopathic and syndrome are therefore an essential part of this process of converting a mystery into an apparently soluble puzzle and as such are not neutral descriptions as is claimed, but symbols of hope and belief. The demystification which western medicine claims does not therefore simply follow from the application of medical science and the beneficial results which may be expected to follow from it, rather it depends on an elaborate structure of belief concerning the inevitable progress of medical science which in turn relies on the central assumption of a unified and objective medical system referred to at the outset. Once this is understood as a belief, western medicine no longer has to be accepted as the only certain and exclusive system, nor does the notion of mystery as hidden matter have to be emasculated by being transformed into a series of puzzles. Put another way it is only because of the assumption that western medicine is not a system of belief that it is possible so easily to dispel the notion of mystery, and yet this assumption is itself a belief.

In summary, western medicine deals with mystery as something hidden in such a way as largely to neutralise it, by reducing it to the status of a number of soluble puzzles. There are two ways in which this is maintained, first by claiming that some such puzzles can already be solved and second that the remainder are potentially soluble. These claims are made on the basis of what is seen as a value-free medical science, but in fact they rest on an assumption which embodies a belief system relating to the capabilities of medical knowledge and technology. Then it is only through the denial that this is a belief system that the force of mystery as necessary indeterminacy in medicine can be disclaimed.

There are though, parallel, yet somewhat different ways in which this more complete understanding of mystery has been seen as relating to medicine. These have been conceived through the notion of the 'art of medicine'. It is commonplace to say that medicine is both an art and a science, but great care must be taken in interpreting exactly what is meant by this, because the terms art and science are used in this context in a number of different ways. They are perhaps most frequently referred to in two contrasting manners which are well described by Reiser. He suggests that the first of these was distinguished in the early years of the twentieth century when the role of science in medicine had become well established, and this led some practitioners to take:

> ...pains to distinguish the art from the science of medicine. Through medical science the physician investigated the mechanism of pathology, through medical art he pursued the intricacies of personality; through medical science he studied parts of the patient to find the causes of biological breakdown, through medical art he kept the whole patient together and observed him as he lived and worked. While medical science could be learned from books and in laboratories, medical art could be learned only from experience with patients. Essentially, the argument concluded, the art of medicine was a talent for understanding the human needs of the patient and using this knowledge to manage his illness better.(5)

The interest of these doctors then was in maintaining a sphere of medicine which was separate from its new scientific character and was seen as important enough not to be secondary to it or subsumed under it. This then was the art of medicine which would rank alongside the science of medicine, and would always sustain the traditional aura of medical mystery, by the very fact that it could not be reduced to the scientific rules of rational medicine. In this conceptualisation art and mystery are naturally an important component of medicine.

Alongside this understanding there has developed a second and very different idea of the relationship between the art and science of medicine. Reiser suggests that it began in the following way:

> As the twentieth century progressed, problems that could be dealt with by the art of medicine were redefined in the new psychiatric and sociological terms and gradually brought within the framework of "scientific" medicine through theories about mental and emotional life and social behaviour.(6)

Gordon suggests a rather different but parallel way in which this relationship has developed.(7) She considers that there are two types of medical knowledge and legitimisation, clinical science and clinical expertise (the latter may alternatively be called clinical judgement or clinical experience) and these are linked to the terms 'science' and 'art' of medicine respectively, which are used as two dominant metaphors in medicine. She also concludes with Reiser that clinical science has been and is increasingly taking over from clinical expertise, but not simply through the expansion of scientific methods into new areas. Rather there has been a change in the scientific method itself, involving what has been described as the development of basic clinical science, in an attempt to produce 'a science of the art of medicine'. In essence it depends on a move away from the sole reliance by scientific medicine on the unifactorial disease model, with its direct relationship between each single causal agent and a discrete disease entity, and the introduction of a multifactorial model which depends on the statistical probability of several factors being jointly involved in disease causation. This is a complex process which will be considered in more detail later, in relation to general practice and public health as well as to medical research and the philosophy of science. Its importance for the present is that it appears to connect a range of apparently disparate factors which were not seen as commensurate, into a coherent system which can be unified and objectively described. It therefore claims to provide a mechanism for reducing what was previously an area of indeterminacy into one of increasing exactitude.

These two processes, first the extension of the traditional scientific method to more areas of medicine and second its transformation into a new probabilistic method are both currently employed as accepted and legitimate means of determining the form of true medical knowledge. So although they may potentially conflict with each other they are more usually seen as parallel and complementary developments. What they both provide is a similar view of the relationship between the art and science of medicine, which is no longer one of two separate but complementary parts, but of science increasingly taking over from and displacing the role of the art of medicine.

Seen in historical perspective the medicine of the middle ages could be viewed as consisting of nothing but an art, which science has gradually been replacing and converting into a 'true' system of medicine, as it progresses and expands through more and more discoveries. The end result of this process at some future date, or

at least the ideal, might then be that science will take over entirely from the art of medicine. In the meanwhile the art of medicine would be employed by doctors of necessity, but its status would be diminishing, secondary and inferior to the science of medicine. Hence those who continue to claim that it has a natural and necessary place in its own right are seen as deluding themselves, and by clinging to the art of medicine for its own sake are to be derided as perverse reactionaries in the face of the new medical science. The art of medicine is then no longer being associated with mystery, where mystery is seen as having a genuine place, but with a type of magic or mystique which depends inherently on ignorance and deception. On this view the falsity of magic may have to be employed in medicine because of ignorance of anything better, but there can be no justification for using it except as a last resort, and it must be discarded at the earliest opportunity. Parsons typifies this view seeing the use of magic as an understandable temptation but one which must be resisted whenever possible:
The health situation is a classic one of the combination

> of uncertainty and strong emotional interests which produce a situation of strain and is very frequently a prominent focus of magic. But the fact that the basic cultural tradition of modern medicine is science precludes outright magic, which is explicitly non-scientific.(8)

Clearly understanding the art of medicine as magic depends crucially on the way in which magic is conceived in relation to science as a whole. This latter concern was of great interest to social anthropologists in their investigation of the structure of knowledge in primitive societies at the beginning of the century, and their conclusions have a continuing relevance to our comprehension of the position adopted by western medicine today. Malinowski (following the views of James Frazer) wrote of primitive societies in the 1920s that 'The function of magic is to ritualise man's optimism, to enhance his faith in the victory of hope over fear', whilst at the same time he saw it as having no place in 'our high places of safety in developed civilisation', where he considered it would be both crude and irrelevant.(9) Such a colonial attitude would generally be deplored today and modern commentators see it as not only prejudiced but as scientifically flawed:

> Earlier in this century anthropologists took it for granted that the manifest technological inferiority of primitive societies was the consequence of a general mental incapacity. Belief in magic was a symptom of this inferiority; it provided evidence that all primitive people are essentially childish and mentally confused.(10)

The rejection of such attitudes must then lead to a different view of the role of magic. It can no longer be seen as what Frazer (quoted by Leach) called 'bastard science' whose 'fundamental quality is erroneous belief about cause and effect',(11) or in other words flawed science which required correction. So the basic mistake made by Frazer and Malinowski is now seen as interpreting what they called magic as within the realm of science, whereas the modern view sees it as properly within that of art, where art cannot itself be subordinated to science.

The parallel with the earlier consideration of the relationship between the art and science of medicine is now apparent. Those who view science as gradually replacing art in medicine are in part relying on the same mistaken assumptions as the early twentieth century anthropologists made about magic. First they see the art of medicine as having a place in primitive and past western societies, the latter being regarded as also relatively primitive. Second the art of medicine is viewed as not really an art at all, but false science or magic. Hence this magical element of medicine can be converted into true scientific medicine, but at our present stage of progress residual elements of magic may be an unfortunate necessity. So it is only described as art because of the current lack of something better. Finally, the development from scientific darkness to enlightenment cannot be avoided, so although magic is seen to have no true or lasting worth yet it is also seen as helping to provide a route to scientific salvation. This led Malinowski to conclude that 'we must see in it (magic) the embodiment of the sublime folly of hope, which has yet been the best school of man's character'.(12) Hence magic becomes a kind of blessing in that it is seen as enabling progress through scientific struggle, even though it is counterfeit and so foolish in itself. The art of medicine may then come to be considered in the same way. By way of contrast the modern anthropological view would be to reject this conceptual scheme which runs magic and art together as pseudoscience because it is both prejudiced and theoretically problematic.

It can be seen that the original delineation of medical mysteries as puzzles, which are either already soluble or potentially so, has been converted into the art of medicine viewed as substitute science or magic. These are simply different means of describing what is essentially the same idea that medical mystery or the art of medicine represents an effort to compensate for incomplete knowledge. As a complete account of medical mystery, this view cannot be sustained though because it depends on a belief in the neutrality and hence supremacy of a particular concept of scientific method which is unwarranted. The features of such a position were outlined at the beginning of this chapter, and expressed as they are here could be called a full-blown positivist conception of science, in that the goal is not only seen as discovering objective medical knowledge, but as establishing that this knowledge is all-encompassing and exclusive. Hence there is no room for any component of medical knowledge which does not conform to this conception of science.

There remains the second way of regarding the art of medicine described above which retains a separate sphere for it, alongside the science of medicine. This appears to preserve a true role for the art of medicine, in which there will be an enduring realm of medical knowledge which is mysterious, in that it deals with matters which are inexplicable in terms of orthodox science.

Such a division of knowledge raises two serious difficulties for our present purpose. First if medical science is constantly advancing, the art of medicine may appear to be at best static and at worst marginalised as science takes more and more of the limelight. There is a danger then, that if medical science becomes the overriding focus of what is seen as important in medicine, the art of medicine is diminished and is seen as representing inferior knowledge when compared with the science of medicine. It was earlier described how the art of medicine first became defined as a separate sphere by those who sought a means of defence against the advance of scientific medicine, but because they put forward no positive argument in favour of the art of medicine the initiative was lost to science from the very beginning. Beyond this it also determined that there would be an inevitable opposition between the art and science of medicine, with the two spheres being defined without any means for determining their proper limits or the relationship between them. The idea of antagonism is therefore built into such a system, and in theory the art of medicine has consistently been perceived as the loser throughout the present century (although medical practice reveals a different story which will be discussed later). On this view the charge against the art of medicine is not now of compensating for incomplete knowledge, but the apparently less damaging one of inferior knowledge. However, the effect may be little different, because whereas in the former case the art of medicine was viewed as gradually disappearing in the latter it can simply be ignored and allowed to wither away as unimportant.

This leads to a second difficulty that medical science is not itself to be challenged, but is to continue to retain the status of being value-free and objective. Although the art of medicine is to remain it is not to impinge on or alter the way we perceive medical science. This formulation of the relationship leaves the art of medicine exposed, because it may be attacked by the canons of science but cannot retaliate. It offers an apparently less imperialist and therefore more restrained form of the positivist conception of science than the full-blown variety previously described, but it involves positivism nonetheless, because it is still the unquestioned and unfounded assumptions of value-free knowledge which predominate. The only difference is that there is a possibility of the art of medicine continuing albeit marginally, and there is no guarantee that it will survive at all. So whilst relegating medical mystery to a separate sphere of art may initially appear more attractive than mystery as a puzzle or as substitute science, on closer inspection it is equally flawed.

The two ideas of medical mystery and the art of medicine so far considered as being either definitely expendable or possibly so are not acceptable, because they both reflect the values of the positivist conception of science which presents an oversimplified and incorrect view. Nevertheless positivism has been the dominant influence determining the relationship between medicine and science, and medicine has been immune to many of the theoretical criticisms of positivism which have been developed by philosophers of science from a variety of different perspectives. One way of exploring this issue is by comparing some contemporary works in the social sciences, which demonstrate certain parallels which medicine. Douglas in her celebrated book *Purity and Danger - An Analysis of Concepts of Pollution and Taboo* provides some fruitful insights. What she proposes is that there are always contradictions in society which threaten disorder, but that man constantly strives to establish order, which is symbolised by purity, and 'that rituals of purity and danger create unity in experience'.(13) So that although knowledge and experience are no longer seen as automatically unified, a new element, ritual symbolism, provides the possibility of integration and hence control.

A number of authors have applied a similar form of analysis to medicine, and Posner's work on diabetes as a system of medical control exemplifies this. She suggests that:

> ... the symbolic level of medical reality expressed in ritual and ideological form, is not simply an imperfection left over from a less scientific and rationally-oriented culture, but an integral aspect of our medical culture ... The symbolic mode allows medicine to proceed as if it were more certain, as if its prescriptions were necessarily accurate and scientifically based, and as if the application of medical technology will necessarily achieve its aim. ... In the face of ambiguity and uncertainty it provides a means for medical practice to proceed with clarity and precision.(14)

The problem with this type of analysis though is that symbol and ritual are not being seen as a means by which to describe or illuminate the ambiguity and uncertainty that is considered an inevitable part of medicine, but as a way of managing it. This is achieved through the introduction of a symbolic mode which mediates between different 'levels' of knowledge and practice and so unites them in a coherent whole. 'The symbolic level of medical reality linked the clinical practices, the ideological prescriptions and the belief in the desire for successful control'.(15) The metaphoric description and use of these different 'levels' would seem then to be a device which holds out the possibility of unity, whilst ultimately leaving the positivist pretensions of medical science undisturbed.

Although a different and more satisfactory understanding is being sought, it is constrained and so distorted by the accepted anthropological method. My concern with this is that although symbol and ritual appear to be associated with mystery as an integral part of medicine, integral is being used in a restricted sense. It is being taken to mean necessary in the performance of a particular positivistically conceived view of medicine and not as involving the permeation and so reconceptualisation of the whole of medicine. What Posner seems to be proposing is that the art and science of medicine both retain their own reality at different levels and their own absolute role and meaning. But this state leads to uncertainty which determines that another distinct element the 'symbolic' is required if they are to be held in a new sort of unity which will provide a stable co-existence. Symbol and ritual do not then refer to mystery but are seen as a new mechanism for coming to terms with uncertainty. This mechanism provides a way of ensuring the continuation of both the art and science of medicine, but it does not challenge positivism in relation to either of them. Hence it is not that symbolism challenges our notions of clinical reality, but that clinical reality can be made more complete by the addition of symbolism.

This formulation of the art and science of medicine is then one in which different varieties of accepted medical knowledge can apparently exist in harmony, although each is seen as valid. There is no longer one system of absolute knowledge, so that judgements cannot be made between different levels of knowledge. Symbolic reality becomes one element of this system of knowledge, which plays a key role in making this diversity of true knowledge possible. It is therefore seen as having definite existence which can be completely described, at least in theory, by the methods of the social sciences. Nevertheless this symbolic level of reality is located in a logically ambivalent position and in consequence is frequently referred to as being magical or like magic. Even though it is no longer seen as involving substitute science, the way in which it might operate is unfamiliar and not readily apparent. This ambivalence would appear to arise because of the paradox of the recognition of medical mystery as something involving indeterminacy at the same time as its containment and neutralisation through the designation of a new category of symbolic reality which is invested with the power to mediate between different 'levels' of knowledge. The mysterious has thereby been reformulated so as to be rendered ordinary and understandable and so no longer mysterious. Indeterminacy has been lost and this affects the art as well as the science of medicine, which are both robbed of the possibility of genuine mystery by being made predictable and thus controllable through symbolism.

Is there then a different and more satisfactory way of conceiving of mystery in medicine? Those which have been considered so far have all relied on positivism to some extent, and one of the principal features of positivism is the insistence on the separability of facts and values, and the primacy given to facts. From this perspective medicine is seen as consisting either of nothing more than facts, or of a primary body of facts with a secondary set of values, which are quite distinct from one another. The sense of mystery being sought cannot be expressed within such a framework, because it is either denied altogether or redefined so as to lose its meaning. (The corollary is that it also produces an incoherent conception of science, and this will be considered later). It must first be recognised that facts and

15

values do not stand in opposition to one another but are intimately related so that they cannot be completely disentangled. The art and science of medicine are not then two separate realms which happen to complement each other, but are necessarily intermingled in some way and to some degree, although exactly how has yet to be specified. Mystery cannot therefore be restricted to the art of medicine, because if it is to apply at all, it must do so to medicine as a whole. So mystery is all-pervasive and has a quality of indeterminacy which makes it in some sense ungraspable and hence not to be fitted within a wholly definable structure.

There are then three main strands which when taken together encompass mystery in medicine. First there is an element of indeterminacy and uncertainty about the science of medicine. Second the art of medicine or medical humanities, including both individual and social aspects, present unique and unpredictable aspects. Third these features of the science and the art of medicine interact in such a way as to make the situation more complex.

Considering these three strands in turn, the problem in relation to science in general has been described by Harré as follows:

> In each era scientists find themselves at a loss, incapable of proceeding deeper into nature. And in each era scientists explain this temporary ending of scientific penetration by a metaphysical theory in which what is basic for one time is elevated to the status of the ultimate(16)

The acceptance of positivism in medical science would seem to fit this description, and so despite its technical successes, prevents a more adequate understanding of medicine. Even in the hardest of sciences there must always be radical uncertainty about the status of current knowledge, if only because the extent and boundaries of that knowledge are themselves unknown. Different and wider contexts, which may recast the present enterprise, are always potentially available.

In relation to the art of medicine the problem of acquiring exact and determinate knowledge is even more problematic. As Ryan comments, Aristotle was:

> ... impressed by the multiplicity of different natural phenomena, insisted that we ought only to aim at the kind of exactness which the particular subject-matter permitted, and that it was folly to erect anything grandiose on the weak foundation of our social knowledge.(17)

Ryan then goes on to conclude in relation to the social sciences that:

> It remains true that as a matter of logic, there is predictability in the sense that *if* the same circumstances and antecedents appeared again, and *if* the same causal laws operate, then the same effects will occur. But methodologically,

there is no room for the pursuit of prediction in this sense, since we know that as a matter of fact the same laws will not operate in future and the same initial conditions will not recur.(18)

So as Toulmin argues behavioural rules cannot be regarded as a subspecies of natural laws and:

What principles are relevant to our understanding in any particular case, what terms are at home in our explanations, depend on the context and purposes of our discussions, and so on the complexity of the relationships we have in mind.(19)

Where what is being considered involves the personal and social relationships between health care professionals and patients, which by their very nature are unique, any attempt to reduce them to scientific principles must fail. One important aspect of this is that the responses of all the participants to a situation are constantly being revised, as their feelings, beliefs and judgements alter in relation to each other. So, as with human and social responses in general, the art of medicine is concerned with that aspect of the subject where precise prediction is impossible.

Hence in different ways and to different degrees, indeterminacy is an inevitable feature of both the art and science of medicine, and the importance and complexity of this is magnified once it is accepted that they are not two self-contained and separable aspects but are themselves intimately connected. The notion of mystery in medicine then takes on a deeper significance.

In order to conceive of mystery in this way we must first be prepared to overturn the central assumption of the western tradition described at the outset of this chapter, because a unitary system does not allow for any necessary indeterminacy. It then follows:

... that there may be a collision between ultimate values with no means of rational arbitration between them, and the consequent conclusion that there is no one single path to human fulfilment, individual or collective, has proved deeply disturbing. It entails that the need for choice between ultimate, conflicting values, far from being a rare and anomalous experience in the lives of man, is in fact an intrinsic element in the human condition itself.(20)

It is the disturbing nature of this understanding that has made it so difficult to contemplate, and has led to the different formulations that have been attempted in redescribing and thereby denying the issue in relation to the western tradition in general and western medicine in particular. Birth and death, and illness and disease which fall within the compass of medicine are some of the most disturbing and threatening events in our lives. So for man to desire and to seek certainty in comprehending and dealing with them is readily understandable, but to persist in doing so can lead only to false conclusions and unrealistic expectations, because it will inevitably result in the distortion and mischaracterisation of both mystery and medicine. The explicit recognition of both the universality of mystery as well as the uncertain quality of medicine are therefore essential first steps in ensuring that neither mystery nor medicine lose their true meaning.

This chapter has sought to elucidate the role and meaning of mystery in its relation with medicine. What has become clear is that it is not an issue which can be separated from any aspect of everyday medicine, either in theory or in practice, but rather is an inextricable part of it. Therefore, it has relevance to all aspects of medicine, from the relationship between patients and health care professionals, to the organisation and justification of health-care systems, and to medical epistemology. No dimension of medicine remains untouched by mystery and the main purpose of this study will be to explore many of the consequences which follow from this. But before doing so it may be helpful to gain an understanding of how the present tradition of western medicine has come to put the notion of mystery aside. The next chapter will therefore examine the historical development of western medicine in this respect and how it has led to the contemporary interpretation of mystery.

3 Medical mystery in decline?

T his chapter will seek to analyse the way in which western medicine has come to view itself as developing so as to be rid of mystery through an ever-increasing reliance on scientific rationalism. This process has come about through the historical emergence of what in the twentieth century has become the accepted and traditional medical model based on a positivist conception of science. Questions will then be raised as to the adequacy of this historical interpretation and some neglected aspects will be considered which suggest the need for a re-evaluation of the contemporary understanding of the role of mystery in medicine and whether it is really disappearing.

A fruitful method of exploring how those who presently adhere to the traditional medical model understand it, is to determine how they describe its historical roots; what aspects of medical history they highlight and give credence to as important in their own perception of the contemporary medical scene. Historians see such accounts as inevitably being biased, because they entail assumptions about the status of all past knowledge, as if there were a predetermined thread leading to present-day concerns, so endowing that knowledge with a significance which it could not have had originally.(1) Such work is therefore incapable of providing a plausible understanding of historical events, but by the same token is invaluable as a means of analysing the dominant assumptions underlying medical theory and practice today, and of the assumed route by which they have been derived. This path will therefore be traced as a means to comprehending the perceived historical relation between medicine and mystery.

Contemporary medicine most commonly identifies its true origin as beginning in Ancient Greece, and with the writings of the Hippocratic Collection in particular. Porter describes the general background against which health was understood by Plato:

> Plato explicitly developed the analogy between the hierarchial ordering of the
> healthy soul (in which reason lords it over the base and unruly passions) and
> the organic social order, in which rational guardians possess true authority,

disciplining the anarchic multitude, who have no potential for self-control, but are slaves to their own appetites.(2)

And Dubos comments on Hippocrates as follows:

Hippocratic writings occupy a place in medicine corresponding to that of the Bible in the literature and ethics of Western peoples ... The immense and lasting prestige of his (Hippocrates') writings is due in part to the many - faceted aspects of their message. As in the Bible, again, everyone can find in them something relevant to his preoccupations which has never been stated better and more succinctly.(3)

But what is it that the current medical establishment has chosen to take as significant from Ancient Greece? Plato's legacy is that 'For two thousand years afterwards, healthy minds, healthy bodies and healthy societies were associated with the rule of reason ...'(4) whilst '... Hippocrates stands for rational concepts based on objective knowledge and for the liberation of science in general, and of medicine in particular, from mystic and demonic influences'.(5) So the identification is above all with rationality and reason to the detriment of the non-rational and irrational as conceived within positivism, and this is shown in several expressions of Greek medicine which are highly admired today.

The first is that Greek medicine provided a particular view of medical knowledge involving a unitary medical theory (sometimes called naturalism) to which all medical experience was to be related. Second this all-embracing medical system provided a uniform expression of health and illness complemented by an ontological view of diseases as specific entities. Finally this allowed for detailed empirical observation which is seen as both of practical use, and as the basis of a 'scientific' outlook. These are then the interlocking elements from which Greek medicine derives its hallowed status in contemporary thinking, as they relate to medical knowledge and science.

However the idealisation of Hippocrates goes beyond this because the Hippocratic Oath details ethical principles which have been equally influential in shaping the norms of western medicine to this day. As Jacob observes: 'The Hippocratic ideal is therefore broad enough to encompass ideas of experimental science, patient-centred but doctor-directed medicine, a guild approach to practice and knowledge, and in large measure each of the modern approaches to health care'.(6) So all aspects of medicine are seen as having common roots in Ancient Greece and it is not surprising that the age of Hippocratic medicine is frequently identified as a golden era to be viewed with some nostalgia.

The period of the Roman Empire which follows is not seen as developing anything very distinctive in medicine, but rather as reworking and continuing what went before. So the Romans are sometimes described as the heirs of Greece, particularly through their acceptance of Galen's teachings. It is significant that Galen was Greek but practised in Rome, so that he provided a bridge between the two cultures, and his name survives as the second great medical figure of ancient times, alongside that of Hippocrates, not so much for having introduced anything conceptually new or important, but more as '... the philosophical organiser of medical doctrine for his own time and for later ages.'(7) Hence as far as medicine is concerned the two periods, Greek and Roman, are often run together and described approvingly as Greco-Roman or simply as the Ancient World.

The many centuries which followed, lasting from about A.D.200 to A.D.1500, have been portrayed as starkly different from the utopian image of the Ancient World. Their common description as the 'dark' ages of medicine is illustrative of how they are viewed, being represented as both regressive compared with what had gone before, and the antithesis of everything that is to be valued in modern medicine. Views such as the following, which appears under the revealing heading 'The period of depression in Europe', are still widely held though they are less frequently expressed today:

> The centuries that followed the death of Galen exhibit progressive deterioration of the intellect. For that deterioration many causes have been assigned. An important factor was certainly the philosophical outlook of later paganism. Men lacked a motive for living. Their view of the world was dreary and without hope.(8)

Such backwardness was seen as deriving from and being dominated by a rigid interpretation of Galen's ideas which became known as 'Galenism', a system under which a number of features were developed which are now particularly denigrated. These are a diversity of medical practice; a slavish reliance on medical theory allied to a lack of precise observations in anatomy, pathology and clinical practice; and a belief in spirits, mysticism and religion as the underlying causal explanation of health and illness. Such perspectives are now commonly regarded as irrational because they rely on supernatural rather than natural explanations and are not therefore considered to be 'scientific'; and they are so at variance with current views that they may be described not just as 'dark' or 'depressed' but even as incoherent or the product of a deficient mind.

In fact the fundamental concepts of medical theory and practice during this long period are so alien to modern medical thought, that a description of them reveals an almost perfect mirror image of those of today, and raises the important issue of the place of mystery. Before 1500 there was a sense of mystery entailing man's inability to hope completely to control medical matters which was pervasive and taken for granted, even though it might be envisaged in a variety of different ways.

Hence diversity and competition in medicine were taken to be inevitable and not something that might be overcome in the future. So a great variety of types of practitioner flourished, without any common standard by which to compare and judge their respective merits, and perhaps it is this above all which leads to the contemporary charge that the period was dominated by the irrational and was 'non-scientific'. This apparent failure to justify medical practice led to a distinction being drawn between two very different types of practitioner, both of whom were to become scorned for their lack of 'science'. One relied on elaborate medical theory from which he claimed to deduce the principles by which to practise, but without an experimental method for testing their merits. The other was the practitioner who relied on no theory at all, and became called the empiric, trusting instead to using his remedies by trial and error, depending on how each patient responded. In both instances the place of theory and practice is now viewed as flawed because of the centrality of mystery which is seen as excluding science.

Many of these ideas and practices continued to influence medicine after 1500, but the period from about 1500 to 1800 is seen nevertheless as dramatically different from what went before, being part of the Renaissance and the Enlightenment. The 'dark' ages of medicine, the time of mysterious forces, came to be seen as nothing more than a long chaotic interlude awaiting the reawakening of proper medical theory and practice, to be taken up from where the Ancient World had left off. From this view a long period of medical history can be neatly demarcated and discreetly set aside, as if it comprised an unfortunate lapse in the long march of progress.

However it is only in retrospect that events become interpreted in such a clearcut way and Cunningham suggests that is was Boerhaave (who taught in Leyden) who had a seminal influence in defining the progress of medical history so as to justify the modern view of the eclipse of the 'dark' ages, and especially of Galen's heritage which had formed the basis of medical authority during that long period:

> In the early decades of the eighteenth century Boerhaave created a history whose peaks were Hippocrates, Bacon, Sydenham and Newton. Hippocrates first practised proper medicine. Bacon pointed out the means for its restoration, Sydenham effected its restoration into practice, and Newton provided the (supposedly complementary) means to understand properly the working of the body.(9)

Boerhaave used the ideas of these four men in constructing his own medical system, which was widely adopted in the eighteenth century particularly in Britain, and their significance has been embedded in medical tradition to this day. Thus they have become more than historical figures, being seen as heroes who symbolise different aspects of medicine which continue to be cherished and respected, and their influence will be considered in his light.

The modern view of Hippocrates has already been examined and is seen to contain the seeds which were developed by Bacon, Sydenham and Newton, all of whom were English and were writing in the seventeenth century. The importance of Bacon (1561-1626) is that he is seen as having established the only true ground on which to develop science. He advanced induction rather than deduction, experiment rather than theory, and ontology rather than metaphysical speculation. King has summarised the prevailing assessment of Bacon's contribution as follows:

> The chief elements of modern scientific method we find clearly expressed in Bacon's writings. He demanded observation, experimentation, precision, and cautious generalisation; he recognised the need for controls, the dangers of hastily drawing conclusions, the importance of recognising and overcoming bias, the need for verification, the return to particulars once the generalisation has been made. Bacon had drawn, if not a blueprint, at least careful preliminary sketches for what eventually came to be known as the scientific method.(10)

This estimate of Bacon's position and status has also enhanced the credibility of some of the earlier pioneers of the Renaissance, of whom Vesalius is probably the most revered in medicine today. Vesalius taught in Padua and his most celebrated work *The Fabric of the Human Body* was published in 1543. Its significance lies in the accuracy of his original observations and illustrations, which were taken from Vesalius' own dissections of the human body. Previously reliance had been placed on the authority of Galen's texts, which contained many inaccuracies because they had been derived by inference from dissections on animals. The status that this work with its new spirit of enquiry has acquired has been described by Singer and Underwood:

> The masterpiece of Vesalius is not only the foundation of modern medicine as a science, but the first great positive achievement of science itself in modern times. As such it ranks with another work that appeared in the same year, the treatise of Nicholas Copernicus entitled *De revolutionibus orbium coelestium* ('On the Revolutions of the Celestial Spheres'). The work of Copernicus removed the Earth from the centre of the Universe; that of Vesalius revealed the real structure of man's body.(11)

This link with the wider scientific endeavour was also of great importance in Boerhaave's inclusion of Newton (1642-1727) in his list. Newton's significance has come to be regarded as two-fold. First he developed a physical system of science, which claimed to be unified, absolute and objective, and therefore to be capable of explaining all scientific phenomena. So Newton embodied the ideal, of a single scheme of knowledge, and medicine embraced this notion in the seventeenth and eighteenth centuries by producing many new theories, each claiming to fulfil that ideal. Although no one theory prevailed at this time, it was nevertheless this view of science which informed the medical world and which was to emerge and become predominant in the nineteenth century, and in the main is still accepted today. The second way in which Newton is seen as important is in providing a mechanistic model of science which can be tested in practice. This promoted the study of the body as a machine (which was also developed theoretically under the title 'Iatrophysics') and advanced and gave credibility to a new understanding of physiology, demonstrated most notably by Harvey's studies on the circulation of the blood, which were published in 1628. The orthodox belief at the time, which derived from Galen and Aristotle, was that blood ebbed and flowed, to and from the heart, but using careful observations and experiment Harvey was able to show that the blood circulated around the body. And the importance of his work has been seen not only as a successful demonstration of empirical scientific method, but also as recasting attitudes towards established medical knowledge and theories. He was regarded as a scourge of the old as well as a harbinger of the new, and so has become another symbolic figure in medicine's heroic pantheon. Singer and Underwood typify this understanding of his place in medical history:

> The knowledge of the circulation of the blood has been the basis of the whole of modern Physiology and with it the whole of modern rational Medicine. The attitude of Galen and Aristotle towards the heart and the great vessels passed into the shadow.(12)

So Harvey is seen as rivalling Vesalius as the founder of modern scientific medicine, but whoever takes pride of place it would seem that any modern list of medical heroes would have to include both their names.

The last of Boerhaave's heroic figures to be considered is Sydenham who has come to be regarded by some as England's greatest medical practitioner. Sydenham was a physician who practised in London from 1656 to 1689, and is now seen as far ahead of his time for the principles which he developed and put into practice. Those which are most applauded are his interest in reforming and improving medical practice through the systematic observation of patients independently of any medical theory in order to find new and untried cures, and his focus on the typical manifestations of disease rather than the individual patient's unique experience of illness. Hence he used an inductive method starting with case-histories from many patients and deriving general accounts of disease from them. Sydenham was therefore the first physician consistently to apply Bacon's empirical methods to his medical practice. He favoured an ontological conception of disease assuming that all diseases are natural discrete entities awaiting discovery, and is considered to have succeeded in having provided precise descriptions of many diseases which had not been distinguished previously, or had been only vaguely described before. Following from this Sydenham is also seen as an important nosologist promoting and contributing to the view that there is a natural disease classification waiting to be compiled as more and more diseases are correctly categorised.

These medical principles were so alien to the traditional physicians of the day, that most of them would have spurned Sydenham as an empiric. However for those who followed his precepts, he was not an old style empiric who refuted rationalism, but was providing a wholly new interpretation of what constituted proper medical practice, one which converted the trial and error of the empiric into an exact method involving disciplined observation aimed at uncovering a natural order. This system offered a revised rationalism which dispensed with abstract theory by claiming that theoretical speculation was redundant, being replaced by observational methods. So the old taunts concerning the respective claims of haphazard empirics and empty theorists were no longer of relevance; they simply had no purchase in the new order. What Sydenham had done, that was seen as of such significance by future medical generations, was to combine theoretical and practical ideas into a new medical understanding, one in which facts were no longer tied inextricably to the patient's illness and his values; and because only doctors were able to elicit and interpret these facts, the relationship between doctor and patient would in future become redefined as well.

Following Boerhaave's elevation of Sydenham as one of his symbolic heroes, these ideas were gradually disseminated and took hold in the eighteenth century, and during the nineteenth century Sydenham Societies were formed in remembrance of his work. Sydenham had come to be seen as a pivotal figure who laid the basis for the modern understanding of medical scientific knowledge, practice and professionalism, in a complete and coherent system combining medical science, practice and philosophy, and it was this that earned him the title of the 'English Hippocrates'. This linkage between Sydenham and Hippocrates had a dual purpose, in that it not only ensured Sydenham a favoured and honourable place in the development of medical thought, but it also involved a reinterpretation of Hippocrates, emphasising those features of the Hippocratic Collection, outlined at the beginning of this chapter, which fitted with the view being taken of Sydenham. This secured the direct relationship that was already being forged between the Ancient Greeks and the seventeenth century, and in doing so further suppressed and denied the ideas of Galenism, which had held sway for some 1300 years.

So by 1800 the outlines of a scheme of medical scientific rationality were discernable, in which facts could stand revealed and the mystery associated with earlier times might one day be a thing of the past. Yet in most respects medical practice in 1800 was little different than it had been in 1600. With the demise of

Galenism medical theory had been transformed between 1600 and 1700, but this had little influence on practice. Jewson's description of the mode of practice (which he calls *Bedside Medicine*) typical of the second half of the eighteenth century illustrates this well:

> The two major growth points of *Bedside Medicine* were phenomenological nosology and speculative pathology. Both activities generated a large number of often mutually contradictory theories, and as a result medical knowledge consisted of a chaotic diversity of schools of thought. The definition of the field was diffuse and problematic, disciplinary boundaries weak and amorphous. The fundamental premises of the subject were a matter of dispute and debate. Rivalry between the proponents of the various theories was commonly conducted at the level of personal abuse and dogmatic polemic.(13)

Bedside Medicine like the medicines of the 'dark' ages was patient-led and diverse, and its practitioners so fragmented and divided as hardly to represent a coherent profession; and all of these features which are negatively regarded today are hardly consistent with the claims of rational scientific medicine.

There were a number of reasons for this. First despite Sydenham's innovations, medical diagnosis continued to depend largely on the case-history and visual observation of the patient. In fact the case-history alone was often considered sufficient, and many physicians conducted a considerable practice by correspondence, both diagnosing and treating patients without ever seeing them. Second and congruent with the reliance on verbal and visual techniques for diagnosis was the employment of phenomenological systems of nosology. These contained vast lists of symptoms which were seen to be naturally ordered, and equivalent to botanical classifications, and were developed and elaborated in the eighteenth century, notably by Sauvages and Cullen. They were so open and non-specific as to accommodate the great varieties of medical theories and speculative pathologies which continued to flourish. Practice was still centred on the patient's home, and the patient paid for attendance and treatment by the doctor. This gave the patient considerable control of the situation, which he was able to exercise by choosing between rival practitioners and the different systems of care which they offered.

The final period to be considered is that from 1800 to the present, the era when rational scientific medicine is finally seen to triumph through the development of a medical model which derives from a positivist conception of science. All the innovations of the earlier medical heroes which had left medical practice largely unchanged, are seen at last to come together and with additional medical insights to form a coherent and comprehensive medical scheme, which fulfils the promise of Sydenham's work to unite medical knowledge, theory and practice. How though was this transformation effected?

It is now conventional wisdom that the most significant changes occurred in the Paris Hospitals during the early years of the nineteenth century. Foucault has been most influential in establishing the idea that there was a crucial change in medical conceptualisation at this time. In *The Birth of the Clinic* he dates it precisely to the year 1801 when Bichat's work *Anatomie Générale* was published: '... the great break in the history of Western medicine dates precisely from the moment clinical experience became the anatomo-clinical gaze.'(14) The sick patient is no longer seen as the primary focus, because attention has switched to the disease defined in terms of underlying pathology. Hence the following line by Bichat is chosen and quoted by Foucault for its special relevance: 'Open up a few corpses: you will dissipate at once the darkness that observation alone could not dissipate'.(15) So for Foucault this new understanding of pathology is the key to the redirection of the medical gaze, and marks a decisive break with the past which heralds a new era in medicine as a whole.

Following the same line of argument Jewson describes this as a threshold between two medical cosmologies (or total systems of medical discourse) that of Bedside Medicine described previously, and Hospital Medicine. He agrees with Foucault in stating that 'The major achievement of the Parisian School was the delineation of objective disease entities by means of correlating external symptoms with internal lesions',(16) and considers that this new conceptualisation was brought about through four great innovations - structured nosology, localised pathology, physical examination and statistical analysis, which were to become the cornerstones of *Hospital Medicine*.

Further important changes which were to alter *Hospital Medicine* occurred later in the nineteenth century and of these two are usually regarded as of most importance. The first began in the German universities in the middle of the century, and involved a move away from gross pathological anatomy to the cellular level, which led to the development of histology, physiology and biochemistry, all pursued within the laboratory. In Jewson's terminology this ushered in a third type of medical cosmology, that of *Laboratory Medicine*, which he suggests led to a switch in interest away from diagnosis and classification, to analysis and explanation, with a consequent shift in attention from medical practice to the laboratory. However, although *Laboratory Medicine* provided the means to much greater scientific understanding of the workings of the body in both health and disease, it did not produce a new understanding of how diseases were caused that would allow the new scientific techniques to be deployed in the search for new and better remedies.

This required a second change, the foundation and application of microbiology which was also dependent on the laboratory. It was this development which enabled the germ theory to be formulated, based on the conceptualisation of microorganisms as specific causes of disease; and it is now regarded as the final and crowning episode that was to place medicine on a truly scientific footing. So it is not surprising that the two men most closely associated with its genesis, Pasteur and Koch, would now be highly acclaimed in any list of medical heroes. Pasteur was the first scientist systematically to develop techniques for studying micro-organisms and to demonstrate their role in a range of diseases in both man and animals. Koch also carried out much practical work on several different organisms, and his most celebrated discovery is probably that of the role of the tubercle bacillus in 1882. But he is equally well known for his theoretical work on his postulates, which provided a scientific framework giving substance to the germ theory and laying the groundwork for the more general unifactorial and multifactorial theories of disease which were to form the foundation of medical theory over the next century. These postulates were a set of criteria for establishing whether a specific organism caused a particular disease. They had their origin in Henlé's theoretical work published in 1840,[17] but Koch's definitive article did not appear until 1891.[18] However the logic of the postulates was implicit in Koch's earlier practical investigations, and these two linked achievements, one in medical practice demonstrating the cause and the hope of a cure for tuberculosis, the greatest medical scourge of the age, and the other in medical theory, received enormous acclaim from doctors and the public. It seemed like a new era as this passage from a textbook of 1883 shows:

> No other event in the history of the investigation of disease has at once attracted such universal attention and interest as did the announcement by Dr Robert Koch, in 1882, of the discovery of the bacillus tuberculosis. The alarming prevalence, the obscure origin, and the almost invariably fatal termination of tuberculosis, render a better knowledge of it most highly desirable.[19]

Also by this time, the focus of medical attention and prestige had become firmly associated with the hospital and its attendant laboratory technology. So the latter part of the nineteenth century can be seen as the period when a particular rational view of medicine became truly established. It was based on a positivist conception of science expressed in a reductionist and mechanical model of medicine, which became widely recognised as medicine's true path and its hope for the future, and has largely remained so ever since.

This new image of a positivist and reductionist model of medicine and its intimate ties with the hospital has been reconstituted and reinforced in the twentieth century in a number of different ways, which have been both a consequence of the model's applications, and an enriching of its theoretical structures to deal with changing circumstances. Four developments which have been of most relevance to this process, and which are interrelated are:

(1) the ever-expanding growth and range of new medical techniques, which have

enabled the extension and refinement of clinical investigations and of disease causation, as well as the discovery of new drugs and other therapies;

(2) the application of scientific methods of assessment to all medical procedures. These are now considered a standard part of good medical practice, whereas they were rarely employed a century ago, and this change has depended on the development of other techniques, especially those of statistics and more recently computing;

(3) the expansion of the germ theory of disease, first to encompass a wider range of causes under the unifactorial model, and second its conversion into the multifactorial model allowing the inclusion of a number of causal elements in a single disease. The latter has evolved more recently as the burden of ill-health in the population has shifted from communicable to non-communicable disease. However the conceptual basis of the multifactorial model is little different from that of the unifactorial model, and the two models are not seen as competitors but are operated in parallel;

(4) the ontological conception of disease which continues to provide the underpinning for an ongoing medical consensus, and so the discovery and refinement of diseases and the consequent updating of disease classification as an important task. The universality with which this is seen to apply is perhaps best demonstrated by the International List of Causes of Death which originated in 1893. After many revisions in the twentieth century, it is now known as the International Statistical Classification of Diseases, Injuries and Causes of Death (ICD) having been enlarged in scope to include morbidity as well as mortality data, and is currently used throughout the world.

These changes may all be seen as appropriate responses to the interpretation and application of the traditional medical model which had been defined by Koch. None of them has been regarded as presenting challenges to the model, whose basic assumptions have therefore remained intact. So all the technical medical advances and changes in health care systems and practice of the twentieth century have become represented as a flowering of principles laid down a century ago. What has not been involved is any serious questioning as to whether this has been the best route to follow or doubt as to the moral and scientific basis on which it has been built. The process has been enabled by the claim that empirical scientific rationalism as applied to medicine is value-free, and that the forms of medical knowledge and practice which flow from it are therefore given. As a corollary, uncertainty and mystery have no place in this scheme, and as history unfolds it is presumed that they will gradually be eliminated. And this process is seen as inevitable, with the way forward being presented as morally neutral.

This representation of medical history may now be summarised as follows. Medical history is a process of development through the emergence and progress of empirical scientific rationalism, especially as embodied in the medical model which contains the ontological concept of disease. The philosophical background to this development has occurred in two stages, first that of the Ancient World (Hippocrates and Galen), and second that of the Renaissance and the Enlightenment (Vesalius, Bacon, Harvey and Newton). The disease concept which followed has three elements and was discovered in three stages between about 1650 and 1875. These are the clinical (Sydenham), the pathological (Bichat) and the causal (Pasteur and Koch). The task now is to re-examine this account and to probe its adequacy, particularly with regard to the perception of its being value-free, and having no place for mystery in medicine.

The history of medicine as presented above is seriously flawed. Indeed it can hardly be described as history at all, because it is not an attempt to interpret and understand the past, but a celebration of the currently dominant medical ideas and beliefs. This is not to deny the need for interpretation, but to question the validity of such an egocentric focus. There are a number of features which demonstrate this, and reveal its weakness. First it is taken for granted that there is a coherent development and upward progress of ideas, which leads to the present and points beyond it to the right way for the future. There is therefore a predetermined selection and interpretation both of the historical periods which are to be considered significant, and the medical figures who are to count. In the latter case those who became identified as heroes of medical history have certain characteristics in common. They were almost always physicians (that is doctors of superior rank) or scientists and so were members of an elite who were accorded high status in their own time. However, typically they did not follow mainstream ideas of their period, and were sometimes regarded as marginal or eccentric figures, their ideas being recognised as significant only later.

So these medical heroes are doubly atypical, not being part of the main body of their contemporary practitioners, and not reflecting the views of their peers. In fact it is only through their contributions being different that they later became seen as being exceptional and heroic. But it is the exaggeration of the differences and the failure to appreciate continuities which reinforces the view that medical history is a positive progression developing in a series of sharply identifiable steps, associated with each medical hero. It appears that these great men advance by making individual breakthroughs and there is little sense of the influence of their colleagues, or of the social and political context within which they worked. Consequently scant attention is paid to the wider perspective, which would encompass the views of doctors and scientists with different approaches, as well as those of other health care providers, patients and the public. This understanding of medical history as the collected wisdom of a few great men has been roundly criticised in recent years by social historians and medical sociologists, but it continues to exert a strong hold on health care practitioners and the public alike. Hence the focus of what is taken as historical medical evidence is for most people still extraordinarily narrow and distorted, and it is this that must be redressed not just for the sake of better medical history, but also and of more importance in this context, as a corrective to current medical assumptions.

At the beginning of this chapter a brief description was given of how Ancient Greek Medicine and Hippocratic Medicine in particular have become seen as the original source of western medicine's knowledge and values. This is fundamental to the comprehension of all later medical conceptions because it has formed the bedrock from which contemporary medicine has developed its most strongly held assumptions. Understanding the limits and deficiencies of the account already given of Ancient Greek medicine is therefore an essential starting point, and one of the most important elements in this is the understanding of health and disease.

Greek medicine contained two philosophical traditions described by Dubos:

> The myths of Hygeia and Asclepius symbolise the never-ending oscillation between two different points of view in medicine. For the worshippers of Hygeia, health is the natural order of things, a positive attribute to which men are entitled if they govern their lives wisely. According to them, the most important function of medicine is to discover and teach the natural laws which will ensure a man a healthy mind in a healthy body. More sceptical or wiser in the ways of the world, the followers of Asclepius believe that the chief role of the physicians is to treat disease, to restore health by correcting any imperfection caused by the accidents of birth or of life.(20)

Western medicine has emphasised the Asclepian point of view and focused on health as the absence of disease, at the expense of the Hygeian alternative of health as a positive general status. Further than this both aspects have been interpreted in relation to Plato's philosophical understanding of rationality, reason and social order. But in Ancient Greece there were contrary strains of philosophical thought which ensured that medicine did not have such certain outlines as may now appear. Today a thoroughgoing rationalist interpretation of the Asclepian understanding views it as ontological, focusing on diseases as discrete and discoverable units, the building blocks from which a secure medical system can be derived. Yet it is doubtful whether within Hippocratic Medicine this ontological conception was so clear, partly because of philosophical diversity but also because the technical knowledge was not available to sustain such a view in practice. Therefore the Asclepian notion formed only one pole in Hippocratic Medicine and was less well defined than is usually suggested, being more consistent with our current notion of medical disorder than with disease, so that normative questions of the meaning of disorder and the proper limits of *medical* disorder were never entirely avoided. In contrast to this contemporary medicine has come to define disease as a more real and distinct notion than disorder, and it is this which has led to a one-sided account of Hippocratic Medicine, with stress being laid on ontology alone.

The idea of disorder provides a link to a consideration of health as order and harmony, the other half of the Greek concept of health as a positive general status which was symbolised by Hygeia. A more satisfactory and complete account of the Greek understanding of health and disease as more than just opposites can then be discerned, through the integration of the two traditions and their respective insights:

> ... Greek medicine, in the Hippocratic writings and practices, offers a conception of disease which is no longer localizationist, but totalizing. Nature (physis), within man as well as without is harmony and equilibrium. The disturbance of this harmony, of this equilibrium, is called disease. In this case, disease is not somewhere in man, it is everywhere in him; it is the whole man.(21)

What emerges from the writings of both Dubos and Canguilhem quoted above, is that although medical thought has always alternated between these two symbolic representatives of health and disease, neither has ever become predominant, and Dubos concludes that 'In one form or another these two complementary aspects of medicine have always existed simultaneously in all civilisations.'(22) Yet this is precisely what western medicine has attempted to deny by claiming that the Asclepian conception should naturally take precedence, and that the Hygeian conception is either not part of rational scientific medicine, or only has a secondary and doubtful role and status. And this attempt to suppress or marginalise the Hygeian point of view has been paralleled by the suppression and marginalisation of mystery in medicine. So it might be thought that the restoration of a system involving a balance between the two poles of Asclepius and Hygeia would also entail the restoration of mystery in medicine. However there is not a direct relationship between the Hygeian conception and medical mystery as can be illustrated by considering the humours.

The rationalist conception of four humours which was originally developed by Aristotle and Galen derives from the Hygeian notion of health as harmony. Strictly speaking there are no specific diseases within this system, only disease processes which are infinitely varied and an expression of disequilibrium in individuals. Hence the patient develops a disease condition as a reaction to ill-health and as a means to getting well. It follows that the appropriate focus of medical care is prognosis rather than diagnosis and on assisting the disease process rather than counteracting it. But this emphasis on health as perfect harmony and on the necessity of ensuring the exact treatment to match the varied needs of each individual patient draws attention to the inadequacy of the physician to the task. With great skill he might hope to restore the patient for a time, but to be healthy is to be constantly at risk of becoming unhealthy, and so can never be securely achieved.

The Asclepian notion of disease ontology would seem to be necessary as a corrective to this untenable abstraction of absolute health, producing a more rounded conception of health and disease. But even this more complete and balanced view, which was characteristic of Greek Medicine, cannot hide the precarious nature of any wholly rational conception. So although the inclusion of the two aspects symbolised by Asclepius and Hygeia does not require the recognition of mystery, it does emphasise that no rational scheme can be stable or sufficient on its own, because it is always vulnerable to other forces. As Porter suggests '... the Greeks did not deny the reality of all that was irrational. Indeed, the very adulation they accorded to reason surely attests to the strength which they attribute to the mysterious forces of passion, of destiny, of fate which reason opposed ...'.(23) It would seem then that excluding the Hygeian notion from any system of medicine, makes it easier for that system to be regarded as securely rational; and the disengagement from the humours over several centuries is therefore one route by which western medicine has attempted to claim such rationality and distanced itself from mystery.

The medical heroes of the seventeenth century who have been previously identified will be considered next, to show that the history of ideas does not proceed via abrupt and progressive changes associated with a handful of great men, but in a more gradual and haphazard fashion. Although humoral theory began with the Ancient Greeks it is also relevant here, because it persisted largely unchanged and was of great influence until its demise in the first half of the nineteenth century. The new spirit of empirical scientific enquiry of the seventeenth century which has already been described as being pioneered by the work of Bacon, Harvey and Newton, was paralleled by work by Sylvius de la Boë (1614-1672) on the conceptualisation of pulmonary tuberculosis. Pagel describes this as follows:

> [He sees] ... his original observation of "glandular tubercles in the lung" as the anatomical basis of cavitation and phthisis. This he feels, should replace the opinion which had been ruling since Hippocratic times, that cavitation was due to a haemorrhage followed by suppuration and decay of the effused blood. Yet ... it is well known how, up to the time of Bayle (1774-1816) and Laennec (1781-1826) de la Boë's discovery was neglected and the ancient theory of cavitation as a sequel to a pulmonary haematoma tenaciously adhered to.(24)

And even later there were those like Andral (1797-1876) who sought to maintain and revive the humoral tradition. So for pulmonary tuberculosis, as with other diseases, the ontological concept described by Sylvius gained acceptance only very slowly over a period of more than two centuries, and during this time many physicians continued to favour humoral theory.

Further than this it must not be assumed that particular medical figures fall neatly on one side or other of such debates. For example in relation to Paracelsus and Newton, Webster has shown that far from being part of two irreconcilable traditions, one pre-scientific and the other scientific, as is commonly supposed, they in fact shared many ideas in common, most notably an attachment to prophecy, spiritual magic and demonic magic. These were characteristic of Paracelsus' time (1493-1541) but did not die out suddenly, persisting throughout the sixteenth and seventeenth centuries and having important influences on Newton's work. So there is a real difficulty in the way in which heroes have been created, a few such as Newton having been raised too high, whilst others such as Paracelsus have tended to be ignored. Webster concludes that:

> In reality the world view of the Scientific Revolution should be viewed as a diverse phenomenon, the result of a dynamic interplay of forces which emanated from many different directions. All of these forces contributed to the process of creativity and change, and none of them deserves to be written off *a priori* as a useless intellectual encumbrance from a discredited magical past.(25)

Even the gradual progression of similar ideas can be overlooked by concentrating exclusively on a particular individual. For example Morgagni's pioneering work on anatomical pathology which was published in 1761 was an important development in changing the medical focus, and was a precursor to Bichat's *Anatomie Générale* of 1801. However Foucault's description of the latter work unconvincingly suggests that it represents a sudden change of consciousness, rather than being part of an emerging set of new ideas.(26)

In a similar way the emergence and acceptance of germ theory and the corresponding unifactorial theory of disease in the second half of the nineteenth century did not herald any dramatic changes in medical treatment, because it was only after many decades that significant new therapies were developed. The case of tuberculosis illustrates this well and is instructive. It was not until the 1950s that specific drugs were widely introduced which were active against the tubercle bacillus, and in the intervening years the mortality rates from tuberculosis had declined dramatically unrelated to these theoretical changes, but due to the general improvement in living conditions.(27) So the overall impact of these new treatments, and of the disease model from which they had been derived, was fairly small.

These arguments then show clearly that medical history has not developed by a progressive series of readily identified steps, but this alone does not contradict the idea of the decline of mystery, only the manner in which it is supposed to have declined. To counter the notion of such a decline requires the further argument that the selection and concentration on particular facets of history is itself a denial of contrary trends. This process has already been indicated but will now be expanded and further advanced to show how medical history which has focused on the currently accepted medical model ignores or marginalises all that does not fit with its presuppositions.

The traditional medical model as it exists today gives primacy to four elements - diseases, doctors, hospitals and empirical evaluation. Each of these elements can be contrasted with others which give different perspectives and insights, and some of them will now be described to demonstrate the pervasiveness of such contrary ideas and practices, and the challenge they provide to the dominance of the traditional model. It will further be argued that it is precisely these contrasting elements that demonstrate the mysterious aspect of medicine most clearly.

In Britain the Medical Act of 1858 was an important institutional marker of the emergence of the medical model. It established for the first time a legal definition of orthodox and unorthodox practitioners. Those registered by the General Medical Council were henceforth to be regarded as proper doctors, as opposed to all the others who were consigned to a different and lower status. So major areas of practice such as homeopathy, osteopathy, herbal medicine and spiritual healing, which have been consistently resorted to by many patients, are commonly ignored in considering the role of medicine and health care. An important element of this is that unorthodox or alternative medicine is frequently not amenable to empirical scientific evaluation. Indeed if it could be so evaluated this would be one route to its being redefined as orthodox. This division of medicine has therefore consigned all types of practice that don't conform to one mode to the second rank, where they are considered to be of doubtful validity.

Within the accepted and superior medical tradition there are also further divisions and rankings. Towards the end of the nineteenth century the three branches of medicine which are recognised today became firmly established. These are hospital medicine, general practice and public health and are ranked in that order respectively. Hospital medicine is above all associated with the dominant disease model and with the subordination of patients' accounts of illness to the doctors' definition of disease. In contrast general practitioners operate with a system which has been described as biographical medicine, in which patients' accounts of illness and the personal understandings of their meaning receive greater attention.(28) The question then is one of the role of disease compared with that of illness, and whilst in general practice there is more attention to illness, the general orientation towards hospital medicine and hence the narrow medical model remains the dominant if disputed force. Public health raises the more general issue of health as opposed to disease, and of the limits of medicine in influencing health, and so of the need for medicine to address itself to wider questions than simply disease as it affects individuals. Hence the ancient symbol of Hygeia is embodied in the theory and practice of public health. This may lead first to an emphasis on prevention rather than cure, but also to further difficulty in attempting any absolute definition of medicine and medical need. By the criteria of the dominant medical model the issue of where medical concerns end and social and political ones begin is assumed to be unproblematic, and this inevitably makes the inclusion of public health as part of medicine a difficult accommodation. Not surprisingly public health has been made subordinate, yet its influence in improving the health of the population has been enormous. The status of public health may be low, but it is perhaps the real unsung hero of modern medicine.

A different aspect of the current medical model is the emphasis of doctors and hospitals on acute conditions and their cure rather than on chronic conditions and care. However the greatest burden of ill-health arises from the latter. Mental illness, mental handicap, physical handicap and conditions of the elderly mainly require long-term caring, and even acute conditions involve caring as well as curing. Within the health service nurses and many paramedical workers, occupational therapists for example, are most closely involved with such longterm caring, and they constitute the greater proportion of all health care workers. But despite the overwhelming importance of this work and its integral place in medical practice the role of these workers ranks second to that of the hospital doctor. Beyond this there is the great army of lay people who provide longterm support and care to sick relatives and friends. Caring for sickness and the relief of suffering have simply not been accorded the status of diagnosis and cure, yet they are arguably the most fundamental aspects of medicine and health care. So this is another major contrary trend to the perceived dominance of the medical model, and despite recent attempts to suggest otherwise, the nature of care is such that it is not wholly open to empirical evaluation. Compassion and trust, which are central to the notion of care and the relief of suffering, can be neither quantified nor purchased.

These then are some of the trends which are of great practical significance and challenge the dominance of the traditional model. They emphasise health and illness rather than disease; the main body of health workers rather than doctors; the community rather than hospitals; and the limits of empirical scientific evaluation. It is this last feature of objective evaluation which is the final guarantee of the medical model, and so to undermine its centrality is also to undermine the model.

Given this different perspective, how has the idealised version of the medical model attained such prestige and become so predominant in theory if not in practice? The accepted answer is that it has been successful in promoting medical technology in a way which is objective and is morally neutral and by contrast any activity which does not conform to its tenets becomes viewed as retrogressive or at least of secondary importance. Uncertainty and mystery which are seen to be associated with a range of contrary practices, must be gradually eliminated, or converted to fit the model, or remain subordinate; and through this process it is seen that medical mystery must inevitably decline. But analysis of the trends outlined above suggests the reverse: that because of the failure of medical practice to conform to medical theory and become unified mystery is not in decline. An attempt has been made to hive off mystery so as to bolster the assumptions of the medical model, and in the process it may appear that mystery has been suppressed, but it has clearly not been eliminated. The paradox is that medical mystery thrives throughout medicine, but within a system which seeks to deny it. The failure is of the medical model to conform to practice, not of practice to conform to the medical model. There is no absolute model which can be separated out and held up as a pure standard to aspire to, and the various strategies for dealing with those aspects of medicine which do not conform to one pattern have no solid foundation.

However the consequences of the misapprehensions which have been described have been grossly distorting to medicine and health care, and the way forward should be in the recognition of the place of mystery in every theory, practice and system of health care. The importance of the contrary trends outlined above and the re-evaluation of their place is therefore vital. However this does not mean focusing on them as exclusive alternatives, but rather seeing the need for the reinterpretation and integration of the whole of medicine by taking into account the proper role of both mystery and scientific rationalism.

4 Mystery and some medical critiques

The last chapter explored the relationship between mystery and the historical development of the traditional medical model. It was shown that the claim that mystery has become separated from mainstream medicine and marginalised holds true only inasmuch as this model has become dominant, and though this may be so in theory it is much less true in practice. Nevertheless this theoretical claim distorts practice, so that although mystery continues to be central to modern western medicine, the image is that it is declining. This chapter will therefore examine how a number of recent critiques of medicine would deal with the notion of mystery, to determine whether and if so how far they share these presuppositions. Six critiques will be considered: those of Cochrane, McKeown, Illich, Fulford, Dubos and Cassell.

Cochrane

In *Effectiveness and Efficiency*[1] Cochrane argued that the main criticism to be levelled at modern medicine was its failure to apply the methods of empirical scientific evaluation. His concern was that time and time again new medical procedures and services are introduced and become widely available without their having been assessed. His remedy was therefore to argue that whenever possible a cost/benefits approach should be adopted through the application of randomised controlled trials.

This criticism of the practice of western medicine is not then a critique of the traditional medical model but rather a plea for greater adherence to its tenets. What it does not question is why doctors should be so consistently resistant to the systematic scientific evaluation of their practice. It assumes that this is a matter of educating doctors out of bad habits to more rational ways of behaving. The logic is that medical practice should conform to the traditional medical model and so no question is raised as to whether the model itself is adequate. It is therefore taken for granted that the right way forward is through the elimination of mystery in

39

practice as well as in theory.

McKeown

In the *Role of Medicine*(2) McKeown presents a more thoroughgoing critique than that of Cochrane. He argues that the improvements in the general level of health of the population over the past three centuries, as measured by overall rates of mortality and morbidity, have in the main been brought about through changes that can be related not to the traditional medical model, but to improvements in nutrition, environmental conditions, and the limitation of family size. He illustrates this by a consideration of the historical changes in the pattern of infectious diseases showing that the introduction of specific medical measures in recent years has had relatively little impact on the downward trend in mortality rates. He then draws attention to the neglect of recognition of public health measures as opposed to measures aimed at the reduction of disease in particular individuals. What McKeown highlights is the reality in medical practice of a balance between Asclepius and Hygeia, and the need to accord the Hygeian aspect its rightful place rather than ignoring or suppressing it as the traditional medical model tends to do. So his critique provides a necessary corrective and plays down the significance of doctors, hospitals and specific disease entities. However it is not altogether a denial of the model and in one important respect reinforces it, by requiring that all procedures be subjected to empirical scientific evaluation. It is then above all a rational scientific analysis which meets the traditional medical model on its own ground, and conceptualises the problem as one requiring the enlargement of the scope of the traditional medical model, to bring more factors into its explanatory domain, and not of challenging it head on. Although this introduces a new perspective which represents an important and significant change, ultimately it does not entail a radical departure because as with Cochrane, the project of the elimination of any non-rational or irrational elements is once again furthered, in this case through the adaptation of theory to meet that end.

Illich

Whilst Cochrane reinforced the traditional medical model, and McKeown proposed only a modification of it, albeit a major one, Illich has developed a fullblown and sustained critique.(3) He draws extensively on the material of other critiques and develops a range of arguments not all of which will be considered here. The focus will be on his central criticism that medicine has developed in such a way as to threaten peoples' health by expropriating it, and this he describes in terms of iatrogenesis which he summarises as follows:

> Increasing and irreparable damage accompanies present industrial expansion in all sectors. In medicine this damage appears as iatrogenesis. Iatrogenesis is clinical when pain, sickness and death result from medical care; it is social when health policies reinforce an industrial organisation that generates ill-health; it is cultural and symbolic when medically sponsored behaviour and delusions restrict the vital autonomy of people by undermining their competence in growing up, caring for each other, and ageing, or when medical intervention cripples personal responses to pain, disability, impairment, anguish and death.(4)

For Illich iatrogenesis is firmly associated with the traditional medical model, and is a powerful, absolute and uncompromising force for evil. All of the consequences of the traditional medical model must then be regarded as bad, because Illich does not see this as just a theoretical model which is only partially operated in practice. So it is not that he wishes to de-emphasise the primacy of doctors, hospitals and the ontological conception of disease, but that he wants to reverse the whole process through which they have become in his eyes, the inevitable concomitants of the worship of science and technology.

However the analysis being developed here would suggest that this medical monolith that Illich opposes is itself a myth, even if its image is real enough to lend support to many of Illich's allegations. There simply is no all-embracing and coherent medical culture which must be rejected in total before any new conception of medicine and health care can be considered. Despite its technical successes and the acclaim it has received the advance of the traditional medical model has been fragmentary and limited. Nevertheless Illich proposes to replace what he sees as an absolute, objective and rational view of a scientific/technological medical model, with the opposite: a view of natural health which both derives from and resides in each individual's autonomous expression of his independence. And as Horrobin observes, by doing so '... he implicitly hints that he is looking back to some ideal time in the past when society was perfect and man was in a natural state.'(5) But it must be questioned whether any such state ever existed, and whether it is possible for any individual to derive an autonomous definition of their own health. What Illich has done is to respond to one medical myth, by creating another that reverses all the features of the first. However if his original analysis of medicine and health care was flawed his own proposals developed by comparison will also be prone to distortion.

Imbuing the individual with a vital autonomy sufficient to ensure his own health is not only implausible, but confers grave disadvantages, which seem at least as serious as those it is designed to avoid, although Illich does not see them as such.

Most notably the endurance of suffering and pain becomes viewed by Illich as ennobling in itself, even forming part of the definition of a healthy life: and death is seen as better than a life lived through reliance on medicine. Whilst Illich may hold such personal values, there would seem no good reason for claiming that others should share them. What it entails is a new definition of medicine and health care, which in common with what it replaces claims to be absolute, objective and rational. This represents itself as a new factual account, which just like the traditional medical model, has no place for the diverse values of individual patients. In this important respect Illich is at one with the ideas of those he criticises in seeing no place for mystery in medicine.

Fulford

In *Moral Theory and Medical Practice* Fulford develops a two-stage critique of medicine. He begins by stating that medical concepts are evaluative and his concern is that 'The evaluative logical element in medicine is located not peripherally but centrally,'(6) and he therefore focuses on illness rather than disease, and shows why it is a mistake to pay attention only to mental illness, as if the nature of physical illness was unproblematic. Sedgwick had pointed out earlier that the anti-psychiatrists 'have accomplished the feat of criticising the concept of mental illness without ever examining the (surely more inclusive and logically prior) concept of illness'.(7) With his attention directed to illness, Fulford then goes on to show that positivist definitions of illness must fail. For example Boorse's well known definition depends on defining illness in terms of disease, which is itself defined in relation to dysfunction.(8) But this is flawed because the key notion dysfunction, is not a value-free term. These elements in the first stage of Fulford's analysis are therefore laudable and unexceptionable.

The difficulty for Fulford comes in the second stage of his argument where he attempts to conceptualise the correct understanding of illness and disease. The problem he wishes to overcome is how to allow for the evaluative nature of illness, whilst retaining something of the objectivity associated with disease. In attempting this he introduces a new term, action failure, which is central to his definition of illness and the key to his argument. Action failure replaces Boorse's notion of dysfunction, and it has two components expressed by Fulford as follows:

> from the "action" in "action failure" come many of the general properties of "illness": its special link with persons, its vagueness, its subjectivity and also, because of the intentionality latent in "ordinary" doing, its properties as a value term ... From the "failure" in "action failure", on the other hand, come all the more specific properties of "illness" as a term expressing a particular kind of

value, negative medical value as distinct from moral and aesthetic value.(9)

The claim then is that action failure can incorporate a general evaluative element as well as a specific element, negative medical value. But this leaves open the question of who is to define negative medical value and how it is to be derived. The danger is that in viewing it as separate from moral value a spurious objectivity is being introduced which although starting from the diversity of values customarily associated with illness ends with a unitary notion, not derived from the experience of patients' illnesses but imposed externally.

There is a parallel here with Illich, whose intention was to substitute patient autonomy for medical paternalism, but who in attempting to do so proposed that a particular set of values had to be attached to the former. Fulford's intention is to switch the focus from disease to illness, but in a similar way he also attaches particular unitary values to the latter. What is forgotten in such approaches is that it is in the nature of both patient autonomy and illness that they allow an unspecified range and diversity of values, so that any move to restrict them is to stifle the process that is supposedly being encouraged, and is to return to the very form of argument that is being criticised. The flaw is in attempting the impossible, to incorporate the subjective and personal in an absolute scheme. Fulford relies on action failure to achieve this, claiming that it represents and promotes the true concept of illness, though it appears more like the introduction of a modified concept of disease, to be objectively defined through its connection with negative medical values.

Fulford starts then from a wholly commendable desire to recognise the centrality of evaluation in medicine and to allow its expression through the inclusion of the diversity of human values. Yet, like Illich, he also feels constrained to impose a particular set of values, and so the end result is that he would seem to be seeking a complete and unified scheme which excludes the possibility of allowing for potentially incompatible values.

Dubos

Dubos adopts an all-embracing Hygeian notion of health, viewing it as a state of complete harmony and happiness involving all aspects of life. By this standard he sees that in reality it must be a mirage, which can never be precisely defined or fully encompassed, because there is no final and determinate goal: 'Progress means only movement without implying any clear statement of direction'.(10) The pursuit of health is therefore an inexact and never ending task, and Dubos gives two reasons why he considers that this is necessarily so.

The first of these concerns the nature of medical knowledge. Dubos describes the historical pattern of disease in different societies and shows that it has developed in ways which could not have been predicted. He considers that this is because of the complexity of the natural world in which events do not occur in a closed or limited system, and this makes it impossible to list all the relevant factors and analyse the processes involved. The second reason concerns the nature of human behaviour which is not governed by biological necessity, so that there is an inescapable component of unpredictability in human life. Hence:

> More often than not the pursuit of health and happiness is guided by urges which are social rather than biological; urges which are so peculiar to man as to be meaningless for other living things because they are of no importance for the survival of the individual or of the species.(11)

Further than this Dubos sees these two reasons as being interrelated. Even assuming that the complexity of nature and of medical science was capable of being completely analysed factually, medicine and health could still not be reduced to facts and logic alone because man has a choice about those things which he values which goes beyond mere survival or material ease:

> Among other living things, it is man's dignity to value certain ideals above comfort, and even above life. This human trait makes of medicine a philosophy that goes beyond exact medical sciences, because it must encompass not only man as a living machine but also the collective aspirations of mankind.(12)

Medicine and health cannot therefore be seen in terms of science alone and hence medical knowledge is not self-contained but subject to the wide variation in man's goals and values. It is then this compound of medical scientific complexity allied to the diversity of human values which determines that health is a mirage.

In referring to health as a mirage Dubos never describes it in terms of a mystery, but his understanding is very similar to that of medical mystery which was detailed in chapter one. Mystery was described as involving an inescapable element of indeterminacy which gives rise to uncertainty in both the art and science of medicine, which are themselves no longer seen as discrete categories, and this would seem to equate closely with the reasons outlined above, which Dubos gave for considering health a mirage.

However it could be argued that Dubos' understanding of health as a mirage paints an unduly pessimistic picture which is itself very far from being plausible. This is because it places the whole endeavour of medicine and of those engaged in health care in a hopeless never-ending maze of purposeless striving, and this is far too despairing. There are of course great areas of confusion and misunderstanding in medicine and health care and the focus of this study so far has been to show how this came about and the effects it has had. But this has never been meant to imply that there are not other and better directions to be found. Indeed the main purpose of the analysis has been to provide the groundwork for the development of a more satisfactory understanding of how medicine might be improved. The problem for Dubos is that his definition of health is utopian, relating entirely to the Hygeian aspect of health in a way which is apt to become vacuous in its inclusion of all aspects of life and a complete harmonisation of them. The impossibility of describing such a state in concrete terms, let alone achieving it, is then inevitable. Therefore the terms of Dubos' description of health make it logically impossible for medicine and health care to be either successful or optimistic, because nothing they could do would be open to interpretation in this way.

Dubos does in fact draw back a little from this conclusion - 'At most it can be said that, despite so many disheartening setbacks, the activities of man seem to have on the whole a direction upward and forward which tends to better his life physically, intellectually and morally.'(13) However this nod in the direction of some possibility of communal progress does little to soften the main thrust of his argument, which relies instead on the varying values of different individuals:

> The kind of health that men desire most is not necessarily a state in which they experience physical vigour and a sense of well-being, not even one giving them a long life. It is, instead, the condition best suited to reach goals that each individual formulates for himself.(14)

But this amounts to no more than a myriad of individual accounts and so gives no substantive content to Dubos' nebulous theoretical definition of health. What is missing is first an Asclepian component to the definition to match the Hygeian aspect and second a coherent social dimension. One attempt to provide these two aspects, whilst escaping from the traditional medical model and its positivist assumptions has been proposed by Cassell.

Cassell

The goal of medicine and health care is usually described either in terms of diagnosis, treatment and cure (and sometimes also prevention) of disease, disability and injury (which relates to Asclepius), or of the promotion of health (which relates to Hygeia), or of some combination of these two aspects. Cassell suggests that there is a different and more appropriate goal which has been suppressed by the first of these approaches and ignored by the second. He defines this in terms of suffering and its relief through the process of healing, and begins his book *The*

Nature of Suffering and the Goals of Medicine as follows:

> The test of a system of medicine should be its adequacy in the face of suffering; this book starts from the premise that modern medicine fails that test. In fact, the central assumptions on which twentieth century medicine is founded provide no basis for an understanding of suffering. For pain, difficulty in breathing, or other afflictions of the body, superbly yes; for suffering, no. Suffering must inevitably involve the person - bodies do not suffer, persons suffer. (15)

The focus therefore is changed from the disease to the sick person. This may appear at first to be similar to the redirection described by Fulford in focusing on illness instead of disease. However the difference is that for Cassell the switch of attention remains centred on the sick person, rather than on some further abstraction which continues to be associated with the body, and which for Fulford is described as 'action failure'. Cassell goes on to argue that it is only through an engagement with the patient's experience that the doctor can initiate the process of healing and so go beyond the more restricted process of treating the person's body. This commitment to an involvement with the person produces a basic tension for the doctor though, arising from the division of his attention, on the one hand directed to the person and on the other to the person's body:

> Withdrawal from the patient is rewarded with certainty and punished by sterile inadequate knowledge; movement toward the patient is rewarded with knowledge and punished with uncertainties. The fact remains, however, that to disengage from the patient is to lose the ultimate source of knowledge. (16)

Cassell is suggesting therefore not that attention to disease is unimportant, but that it needs to be understood within the context of the sick person and of suffering, because anything less than this wider view diminishes or emasculates the knowledge that can be gained.

Three important issues emerge from this insight:

(1) that changing the goal of medicine away from an exclusive focus on a disease entity, does not entail dispensing with the Asclepian aspect of medicine, but rather transforms it by incorporating knowledge of disease. This perspective has similarities with the humoral conception where the outlines of disease description are still discernible, but as knowledge to be considered in relation to the potentially inexhaustible variety of different sick people;

(2) that the fullest sense of medical knowledge can emerge only from an understanding of sick people by doctors and other healers, and so cannot be derived solely from an individual's formulation of what constitutes health for himself.

Hence the determination of medical knowledge must evolve as a shared enterprise, arising most intensively from the interaction between doctors and patients, but also from the wider interrelationships involving other health carers and the family and community concerned with health care;

(3) that this deeper sense of medical knowledge can be gained only by exploring territory which will inevitably lead to areas of indeterminacy, which is why Cassell describes the relationship between doctor and patient as mysterious. The further the relationship develops, the greater the knowledge that will be attained, but at the same time this will generate increasing levels of insecurity, which can only be successfully dealt with and so enable the healing process, through a deepening of the personal understanding between the doctor and the patient.

Conclusion

Of the medical critiques considered in this chapter, only those of Dubos and Cassell are consonant with the idea of medical mystery. They provide two very different approaches by starting from the opposite perspectives of Hygeia and Asclepius respectively, but when taken together may be viewed as complementary. Dubos can be criticised for employing a notion of health which is too abstract and general to represent an adequate account of the practice of medicine and health care. Nevertheless it is fruitful in giving expression to the ideas of wholeness and harmony as essential components of a complete and satisfactory definition of health. In contrast Cassell grounds his understanding of the goals of medicine firmly in practice through his attention to the sick person and suffering. The opposite criticism of that made of Dubos could then be levelled at Cassell - that he attends too narrowly to clinical medicine and health care practice, and ignores a wider vision of health. Whilst there is some force in this, Cassell's avoidance of a mechanistic conception of disease tends also to lead him towards a more complete notion of health, although more restricted in scope than that of Dubos. So a meeting point can be found between the critiques of Dubos and Cassell, with Dubos painting on a broad canvas and Cassell relating that vision to the reality of personal suffering in medicine.

What both these authors draw attention to is that the foundation of their critiques depends on a critical reassessment of the nature of medical knowledge and its justification, and this will be the subject of more detailed analysis in the next two chapters.

5 The nature and justification of medical theory and knowledge - issues to be considered

As described in chapter two a positivist conception of science first began to be developed in the sixteenth and seventeenth centuries, and gradually came to be applied to different aspects of medicine until by the latter part of the nineteenth century it had become predominant. Indeed the relationship between scientific positivism and medicine became so strong, that it was seen as the proper basis for describing all medical theory and knowledge. Since then this understanding has been modified but it remains as the central pillar of medical justification. This chapter will therefore be concerned first with the form and implications of the identification of scientific positivism with medicine as it was defined in the nineteenth century; second with the changes that have occurred since then; and third with a critical analysis of these evolving medical conceptions.

There were many diverse influences, social as well as scientific, which led to scientific positivism gaining such decisive ascendency in medicine in the second half of the nineteenth century, but the crowning achievement is usually identified as the triumph of the theory of contagionism in the form of germ theory and the infection model of disease. H.A.M.J. Ten Have has analysed the complex process by which the rival theory of miasmatism was finally vanquished, and suggests that:

> Because of its precise results as well as its explanatory power, the infection-model turned out to be the most powerful paradigm of modern scientific medicine; it still represents for many philosophers of medicine the core of the biomedical model of disease and treatment. This model has come to define the nature and role of modern medicine.[1]

The work of Pasteur and Koch is most closely associated with the development of germ theory as a secure basis for establishing medical knowledge, and Koch's postulates had first been worked out as a theoretical scheme by Henlé in 1840, but were not published by Koch until 1891,[2] following his experimental work which had demonstrated their practical scientific value. They stated that:

(1) the organism is always found with the disease in accord with the lesions and clinical stage observed.
(2) the organism is not found with any other disease.
(3) the organism, isolated from one who has the disease and cultured through several generations, produces the disease (in a susceptible experimental animal).

Importantly they contain the three essential elements of Koch's ideal disease model - the causal agent, the pathological lesion and the clinical syndrome - and provide the basis for the outline of a blueprint from which the traditional biomedical model and a programme for western scientific medicine were subsequently derived. It was a new and complete conception of medicine which embodied the strongest and most clearcut expression of scientific positivism in medicine, and in doing so contained a number of interrelated assumptions which include the following:

(1) medical knowledge is determined by what doctors and other health care professionals associated with them do, and conversely only they know properly how to deal with medical matters;
(2) medical knowledge is scientific, effective in technical terms and value-free. Hence social factors which are seen to involve values are distinct from medicine by their very nature;
(3) health is defined as the absence of disease;
(4) illness is conceived as an imperfect account of disease;
(5) disease is a key conceptual component defined in terms of normal biological functioning and specific aetiology. It follows that diseases are seen to exist as discrete objectively defined entities, and that there is a universal disease taxonomy which is potentially completely discoverable.(3)

Doctors and their associated health care professionals derived a new legitimacy and status from this rational and scientific conception of their role and this has continued to the present, despite some changes to the original notion. It was soon realised that the doctrine of specific aetiology was too restrictive to account for the cause of all communicable and non-communicable diseases. So Koch's original unifactorial disease model was modified to allow for more than one causal element, thus becoming the multifactorial disease model. However this has not entirely displaced the unifactorial model and both models continue in parallel. The multifactorial model is now most commonly regarded as a biopsychosocial model because of its inclusion of psychological and social causal factors as well as biological ones. But this expansion of the model has come to be regarded in two very different ways, both of which tend to undermine some of the assumptions of the traditional biomedical conception. On one view psychological and social factors become subject to scientific positivism, but the problem then is that any area of life may potentially be regarded as medical. For those medical imperialists who wish to expand medicine into new areas there is then no ready check, because there is no distinction drawn between the medical realm based on facts and the social realm based on values. What has happened in practice though is less straightforward, and in the twentieth century some areas of life which were not previously regarded as properly the subject of scientific medicine have become so e.g. heroin addiction, whilst others are tending to be given up e.g. mental handicap. On the alternative view the biopsychosocial model is seen as a means of claiming that not all areas of medicine can be interpreted within the framework of scientific positivism. Wulff for example takes this position.(4) The difficulty with this though is first how to define which areas of medicine should be subject to scientific positivism and second how to justify medicine's claim to other areas which are not subject to scientific positivism.

These differences remain unresolved and the position is far less clearcut than the apparently straightforward conception embodied in the original biomedical model. One reflection of this is that different doctors adopt varying stances. Some remain wedded to the traditional biomedical model, whilst others subscribe to the biopsychosocial model but interpret it in different ways. Some philosophers e.g. Thung have taken a further step in claiming that scientific positivism is not applicable to medicine at all,(5) but this position is almost universally rejected by doctors, either explicitly or implicitly. The difficulty they face is that although the logic of the traditional biomedical model and scientific positivism have increasingly been seen to be inadequate in the description of medical practice in the twentieth century, yet to jettison them altogether appears to involve discarding the whole structure, stability and powerful legitimacy that medicine and the medical profession acquired in the nineteenth century. So many doctors are willing to accept a modified version of the traditional biomedical model in which the role of scientific positivism is weaker, but even if it is not made explicit they see that a central core of medicine which is factual, objective and value-free always remains, as a necessary lifeline to the hard won advantages which from a medical perspective purport to be both fundamental and unassailable. Some of the advantages claimed for this conception are that:

(1) it provides the only proper foundation for the role of doctors and other health care professionals working with them, and so maintains their status. This holds even though the argument is circular, because what is proper and scientific positivism are defined in relation to each other. However it is sustainable only whilst scientific positivism retains a general acceptance or there is ignorance amongst the public of the extent of medicine's reliance on positivist assumptions;

(2) it delineates medicine and medical work in a way which: (a) excludes other

claims to medical knowledge and the practitioners associated with them; (b) defines a limit to medical treatment and care; (c) indicates the boundaries of medical welfare and health policy;

(3) it provides a reassuring certainty for both doctor and patient as to their roles, which is often believed to relieve the sick individual of blame and responsibility;

(4) it channels the development of organised scientific research, by providing disease models which give a clearcut framework and definite objectives for empirical investigation.

Turning now to a critique of the way in which the traditional biomedical model and scientific positivism have developed, Koch's postulates will be taken as a starting point. The central claim being made by Koch was that diseases exist as independent and factual entities which can be objectively defined for all time, and his assertion that there were three elements, the causal agent, pathological lesion and clinical syndrome, was essential to an ideal description of disease which provided the structure of how diseases were to be properly defined. In fact this conception of disease contained a logical confusion which undermined the status which Koch thought it had. This may be demonstrated by considering Koch's own example that of pulmonary tuberculosis, and the way in which definitions of disease in relation to Koch's three disease elements have been developed in practice.

The problem raised by this conception of disease was how to define those segments of the model where the elements do not coincide (see Figure 1). Either they do not represent disease because all three elements are always considered necessary, or they represent a disease or disease-related condition although only one or two of the elements are present. Figure 1 shows that in deciding how to interpret this a hierarchy of the three elements has been adopted that allows the latter course to be followed. Consequently all the segments where the causal agent is present (1-4) are related to pulmonary tuberculosis, and a different disease, sarcoidosis is proposed where there is a pathological lesion without the causal agent (5-6), whilst the clinical syndrome alone is given no particular disease status (7). The postulates themselves do not make this clear. On the one hand they stress the primacy of the organism, but they also refer to the organism as if it is separate from the disease, in which case the other elements should take precedence in the definition of the disease. This ambiguity was appreciated by Virchow as early as 1895 when he described how 'the hopeless, never-ending confusion, in which the ideas of being (*ens morbi*) and causation (*causa morbi*) have been arbitrarily thrown together began when microorganisms were finally discovered'.(6) The clinico-pathological elements in combination and the causal element appear to be defined in a circular relationship which can be broken only by making one or other predominant, and this is what has happened in practice by giving the causal element

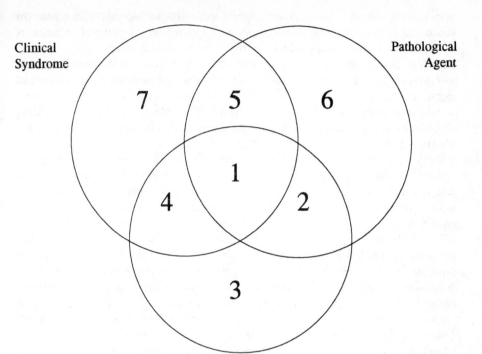

Specific causal agent

Current definitions:

    Pulmonary tuberculosis:
        1. Ideal disease
        2. Subclinical disease
        3. Preclinical disease
        4. Disease - pathology presumed

    Sarcoidosis:
        5. Disease (cause unknown)
        6. Subclinical disease

    Other:
        7. Other clinical disease

Figure 1:   *Development of Western Disease Model as Applied to Pulmonary Tuberculosis*[7] primacy.   However to do so undermines the claim to objectivity, because the process of making that decision requires the introduction of a judgement which in this case involves placing higher values on the causal than on the clinico-pathological elements.   Attempts to deny such use of values may be based on the assertion that the pathological lesion and the clinical syndrome match the causal agent, so that the three circles in the diagram fit closely together.   But such matching is never perfect and any attempt to clarify the relationship actually involves using the postulates as a means of constructing diseases, rather than simply for its claimed purpose of revealing them.   Then because it is impossible that any conception of disease could exclude some element of such construction, the original claims to value-free scientific status as the basis of medical knowledge are undermined at their source.   It is not then just the claim that this is the only way to discover diseases which is false, but the very idea of viewing diseases as specific entities about which such claims could be made.

This did not, however, diminish the importance of Koch's postulates or of the germ theory which underpinned the biomedical model.   There were complex social, political and professional reasons why this was so.   Three important factors will be noted here, because they have continuing relevance today.   The first concerns the optimism generated in the nineteenth century about the possibility of a general science of man, which had been fostered by writers such as Comte and J.S. Mill. They had come to view the relationship of social factors to man in the same positivist manner as was being claimed for the natural sciences.   From this perspective the prospect of constructing theoretical schemes by which to predict and control all aspects of men's lives was seen as a rational development.   The ideological framework which embraced a new model of medicine and natural science was therefore part of a wider set of ideas which both enabled its development and enhanced its credibility.

The second factor concerns the statutory provision of health care.   From the middle of the nineteenth century the state became increasingly involved with providing health services, through poor law hospitals, hospitals for infectious diseases and the mentally ill and handicapped, as well as through a plethora of public health measures.   Much of this reform had been originally inspired by theories of miasmatism and hygienism, but the implications for change and expenditure based on such theories were virtually limitless.   They rested on Hygeian notions of health, where all aspects of life are considered of relevance, and also stressed general environmental forces, rather than individual factors in determining the locus of health and disease.   So these ideas were economically expansionist and threatened the more traditional concern of government, that of curbing and setting limits to public expenditure.

Similar tensions are also evident in Bentham's classical utilitarianism, which had a pervasive influence on all social policy in the first half of the nineteenth century.

On the one hand utilitarianism favoured public investment to improve social and industrial conditions and hence benefit the health of the mass of the people, but government expenditure to achieve this could not be open-ended. Bentham believed that his felicific calculus would set an automatic limit on such public expenditure, because a point would be reached where further expenditure would produce more overall pain than pleasure. But the theory of miasmatism contained no such limiting principle, so there were considerable economic and political arguments for turning away from it.

The third factor which tended to reinforce these arguments for a theoretical redirection was the desire to professionalise medicine, in order to both raise its status and assert its independence. In Britain this was formally achieved through the Medical Act of 1858, which limited those medical practitioners who were henceforth to be considered qualified doctors, by restricting entry to the profession on the basis of education and through a statutory register. The Act also set up the General Medical Council, a professional body internally regulated, and charged with setting medical standards and disciplining its own members. An improvement in medical status and a high degree of independence were thereby achieved and in the process all other practitioners were reduced to a lower rank, offering 'alternative' or 'fringe' medicine. In bringing this about the profession had to overcome two problems. First it had to restrict what was to be considered properly medical. If all areas of life could potentially come under that label, then it would be difficult to claim that only some practitioners with particular knowledge, expertise and remedies should be considered true medical men. Equally if medical men were to determine their own standards and control their own members, they must have an exact and defined body of knowledge which only they could correctly understand and interpret. Miasmatism was deficient in both these respects, being both universal in scope and diffusely structured. In contrast the newly emerging germ theory appeared both to provide clear medical boundaries and to define the special and precise structure of medical knowledge. Further than this in claiming that such medical knowledge was objective, it was not open to challenge from the government, the public or other practitioners. So the implications of germ theory held out many advantages for the profession, but also for the government because of its restriction in scope. In addition it offered unparalleled hope to the general public in its confident claims for the possibility of conquering disease.

Against this background it is perhaps not surprising that though much of government health policy in the second half of the nineteenth century continued to derive from ideas relating to the theory of miasmatism the changes that are proclaimed were mainly justified on the grounds of germ theory. The force of an idea does not derive from its logic alone, but also from the credence which is placed on it, and this relates to a complex of intermeshing social, economic and political interests as well as scientific and professional concerns. The present purpose has not been to explore all these relationships in detail, but to demonstrate some of the reasons why Koch's postulates, germ theory and the now traditional biomedical model became so readily accepted at a particular time in history, despite the logical and conceptual problems which they posed.

The two main conceptual difficulties which have now become apparent are (a) whether diseases are discovered, or derived in some other way; and (b) whether there are any determinate or absolute limits to medicine, health and disease, how they are to be secured, and what assumptions need to be made. The first became apparent from a consideration of the traditional biomedical model, and the second whilst inherent in this model became more explicit when considering the multifactorial, biopsychosocial model. Both these conceptual problems remain unresolved today and will now be considered in more detail.

King poses the question of whether diseases are discovered or created as follows:

> We are faced with the problem whether certain relational patterns, like diseases, "exist in nature", while other patterns, like a melody or a poem, we can create arbitrarily by our own skill and ingenuity. The question becomes, does a disease, whatever it is, have real existence, somehow, in its own right, in the same way as the continent of Australia? Such real existence would be independent of its discovery by explorer or investigator. A disease exists whether we know it or not. The contrasting point of view would hold, that a disease is created by the inquiring intellect, carved out by the very process of classification, in the same way that a statue is carved out of a block of marble, by the chisel strokes of the sculptor.(8)

In the present context the question arises in a particular form - whether positivism or normativism determines the nature of disease. A positivist conception of disease contains two important assumptions, that diseases are defined solely by reference to facts and such facts are naturally determined. Normativism on the other hand, sees the designation of disease as a process involving three principal elements: first that a particular state or condition is judged abnormal; second that such an abnormality is judged to be a disease; and third that some explanation is proffered for such judgements. Whilst positivism claims that diseases are value-free, normativism asserts the opposite, that the whole process of disease ascription is value-laden.

If diseases were derived solely from facts it would be expected that all societies would recognise the same diseases, or where there were discrepancies that these could be resolved by reference to independent scientifically accepted knowledge and when this was deficient to future scientific research. Comparing this with the situation in practice it is quite clear that different societies do not always recognise the same diseases. For example some cultures have viewed what is now considered in the west to be mental illness and disease in religious or magical terms, so excluding it from medicine altogether. Other societies have included conditions within medicine which are not now regarded as medical disorders e.g. the American Psychiatric Association classified homosexuality as an illness until 1974, and in the era of black slavery drapetomania was considered to be a disease which led slaves to run away. Even within a society there are always disputes as to whether certain conditions should be considered medical; a current example in Britain is alcoholism, and new conditions of uncertain status are continually described e.g. myalgic encephalomyelitis (M.E.), and frequently discarded later.

However these variations need not be considered as undermining positivism, if they are seen simply as mistakes which are gradually being clarified and rectified by scientific research. Indeed they may be taken as evidence that scientific positivism is working well in gradually perfecting knowledge of what are true disease categories. But this fails to explain two factors. First why within a particular society, when the facts are well-known, disagreements can still arise, and the example cited of alcoholism fits this description. Second why between two societies there are sometimes opposing notions about a particular disease, although both societies claim to derive their disease categories from the same set of factual medical knowledge. A notable example of this is the designation of low blood pressure as the disease 'hypotension' in Germany, whilst in Britain and most other western countries far from being considered a disease it is seen as a sign of health.(9)

These instances would seem to demonstrate that the designation of disease cannot rest solely on facts and that values must play a part. What part though is not yet clear. A criticism sometimes levelled at those who maintain the necessary involvement of values in all areas of medicine is that this will lead to cultural relativism, a position where simply anything may or may not be considered medical by different societies according to their own internal values. This does not follow though because it would require all societies to have fixed and watertight boundaries across which it was impossible to trespass in making moral judgements.(10) An extreme example of this related to medicine was portrayed by Samuel Butler in his classic fictional work *Erewhon*. He imagined an isolated country where everything considered medical by his own society was seen differently, because the social order was inverted, leaving the usual understanding of crime and disease reversed. Yet as the following extract reveals, to talk of medicine, health and disease at all requires some common understanding of what it should contain:

That in that country if a man falls into ill-health or catches any disorder, or fails bodily in any way before he is seventy years old, he is tried before a jury of his countrymen, and if committed is held up to public scorn and sentenced more or less severely as the case may be. There are subdivisions of illness into crimes and misdemeanours as with offences amongst ourselves - a man being punished very heavily for serious illness, while failure of eyes or hearing in one over sixty-five, who has had good health hitherto, is dealt with by fine only, or imprisonment in default of payment.(11)

For Butler to mention ill-health, disorder and bodily failing must imply some agreed conception of what is involved, and for him to describe those notions as being viewed entirely in terms of crime is to empty them of any comprehensible meaning. This was not a misunderstanding on Butler's part because his intention was satirical, but if his imaginary society were taken literally it would not be that crime and disease were reversed, but that there were no understanding of either of them from within the accustomed frame of reference. It is only the investment of some common values which make crime and disease sufficiently coherent ideas for them to be recognisable.

What is found in practice is that medicine, health and disease are part of a set of ideas about which there is some common understanding within all societies, even though the content varies very considerably. And this is what would be expected, because although there is a common conception, its value-laden nature inevitably leads to a different outline and content in each society, which can never be altogether harmonised. Consideration will now be given to the extent and form of these variations, and how far such variation is morally justified. Despite the substantial differences already noted between societies it would seem unlikely on first consideration that any society would ever consider certain conditions not to be appropriately categorised as medical conditions. Two examples that might fall into this category and will be used as illustrations are broken bones and a fatal episode of heart disease. Those who support a weak form of medical positivism would claim that this is because they are part of a core of value-free medical knowledge, and therefore indisputably medical. But the foundation for such a claim is flawed, because it assumes that such disorders are naturally defined. Boorse, a well-known author in the positivist tradition, interprets this as follows: '... the single unifying property of all recognised diseases of plants and animals appears to be this: that they interfere with one or more functions typically performed within members of the species'.(12) There are two problems with this. First it assumes that each species has a natural design, which is served by typical functioning that is value-free; and criticism of this idea when related to man could be applied to all societies, even those which do not recognise the notion disease, but only a more general category of medical condition or disorder. Second many societies are not principally concerned with technical function in conceptualising medical conditions, but are more interested in establishing the reasons why illnesses should afflict particular persons. So in many traditional societies, a central role of the witch-doctor or shaman is to determine why a significant person or event might have been thought to be the cause of the patient becoming sick.

If however we return to the two examples given of conditions claimed to support this case, it is not the bare facts of broken bones or a fatal heart condition that lead to their being automatically regarded as medical conditions, but the values placed on those facts. The reason that certain conditions are almost invariably considered medical follows because they are consistently valued and therefore judged as falling within a medical category not because there is any strict logical necessity that they be so viewed. Although unlikely it is not inconceivable that any condition could be differently judged as not medical within a particular society. For example in traditional Chinese society girls' feet were tightly bound from childhood to restrict their growth, and this was carried out so forcefully that it led to severe pain with the bones of the feet commonly being broken.(13) The breaking of bones in this manner could either have been regarded as not a medical matter, but as a necessary part of an accepted and normal process, or if a medical matter then not as something dysfunctional or disadvantageous. Similarly with a fatal episode of heart disease, it is possible to imagine a poor and overpopulated society where death in later middle-age became regarded as socially and economically desirable. To aspire to a prosperous life of overeating, smoking and hard stressful work culminating in a swift death from a heart condition at a relatively early age, might then be judged of value and a normal mode of dying not involving disease.

What these two examples, one real and the other imaginary, demonstrate is that there can be no absolute certainty that any particular state or condition will always be regarded as a medical disease or disorder. Social norms within particular societies may determine that particular states are viewed otherwise. However this does not mean that no moral judgements can be made about such social norms (as this would involve an acceptance of cultural relativism), or that any such society could overturn and so dispense with the whole notion of what medicine and health are commonly taken to embody, in the way that Samuel Butler portrayed it in *Erewhon*. It might then be argued that for any society to consider broken bones or a fatal heart condition as not being disorders which fall within a medical category is morally reprehensible, but it would never be possible to resolve such disputes with the same certainty that positivists would claim. Even if in practice it is found that all societies agree about a core of conditions which they consider to fall within a medical category, this is not because there are plain facts which 'speak for themselves', but only because there is a consensus that they should be valued and judged in that way. Furthermore it is certain that such a consensus will never be complete, even over what might have been thought core conditions; whilst disputes over more 'marginal' cases will always be rife. Hence although there must be a universal understanding of a very general overarching notion encompassing health and illness, what that must necessarily contain in any society cannot be specified with precision or certainty either in social or moral terms. The corollary of this is that the significance that conditions considered to be medical may have can be understood only in the context of more general conceptions concerning each particular society.

The claim of positivism to provide a fixed and indisputable account of factual medical conditions, either for all of them (strong positivism) or for a central core (weak positivism), has now been shown to be false. So the advantages traditionally claimed to derive from such a position cannot be sustained. These were set out earlier (see pp.51-52) and must now be revised as follows:

(1) what might serve as an adequate foundation for medical knowledge is not clearcut so the role and status of doctors and other health care professionals working with them cannot rely directly or indirectly on it, there being no absolute knowledge.

(2) because medicine and medical knowledge are open-ended, necessarily incomplete and provisional: (a) other claims to medical knowledge and the status of practitioners associated with them must be re-evaluated; (b) there is no precise limit in defining medical treatment and care; (c) there is no firm indication of the boundaries of medical welfare and health policy.

(3) the basis of both doctor and patient roles is changed. The question arises as to whether the sick individual should bear some blame and responsibility for his condition, although it is recognised that there are aspects of his biological constitution and social circumstances over which he has little control.

(4) the basis of scientific research in medicine is challenged.

Some of these issues will be pursued at length later, but the general point to be made is that although positivism in medicine has proved a very powerful ideological force it has only ever been partially successful in practical terms, and this was inevitable given its own contradictions. So much of the force of the advantages claimed for medical positivism, has been due to the image of medicine which has been presented, rather than to their practical reality. Hence their revision is less dramatic in practical terms than it might appear in theory. Nevertheless the attraction that medical positivism has had and continues to have should not be underestimated, precisely because the image it presents has such strong and appealing resonances for doctors, patients and governments alike. It is this difference between image and reality which has allowed the discrepancies between theory and practice, whilst protecting positivism from searching scrutiny. Although some might see this as unimportant because they regard these developments as essentially benign, this is not so, partly because it is intellectually dishonest, but also because it permits those who are able to harness positivist arguments to their own purposes to do so without being open to proper challenge. So the fact that positivism has had less real influence in medicine than is often suggested, cannot be used as a reason for accepting that its contradictions and distortions continue unhindered. The undoubted attachment to it which there continues to be can no longer be allowed to obscure the importance of normativism with its focus on evaluation and judgement in the provision of a more satisfactory account of medical theory and knowledge.

The assumptions that lie behind scientific positivism in medicine which were outlined earlier in this chapter, should be dispensed with, but the two main conceptual difficulties which were raised still remain. These were (a) whether diseases are discovered or created or derived in some other way; and (b) whether there are any determinate or absolute limits to medicine, health and disease; how they are to be secured; and what assumptions need to be made. Although a different direction has been suggested no answer has yet been given to them, and this will now be attempted. The first point to be made is that in rejecting the role of scientific positivism in medicine it does not follow that facts play no part. The problem is that positivism and normativism are often described as if they were in direct opposition to one another, as are discovery and creation in relation to disease, and it may then seem that there has to be a choice between facts and values in medicine. These are false dichotomies and it is only in attempting to overcome and go beyond them that a more satisfactory analysis of the nature of medical theory and knowledge will be possible.

Three propositions will now be explored which have an important bearing on these questions:

(1) that the purpose of medicine is ultimately concerned with practice rather than abstract knowledge;

(2) hence it is practice and applied knowledge which provide the justification for medicine and give it continuity;

(3) that although there are some similarities, the medical method of theory and practice is different from the more general scientific method.

Medicine is a practical discipline but it also generates its own distinctive theory and knowledge. The problem is to determine the relationship between theory and practice. The positivist conception of medical science views theory and knowledge as an independent realm which can be studied and investigated in isolation from practice and then be applied to it. The opposite view is that practical concerns shape theory and knowledge:

In the applied sciences, epistemic goals are important but non-epistemic goals are central. One frames understandings of the world within an applied science such as medicine not in order to know the world truly, but in order to control the world easily and cheaply.(14)

However it is not the case that either theory or practice has to take precedence, rather that practice and knowledge appropriate to it, proceed hand in hand. So there is no pure or untainted knowledge which provides the definitive justification for practice. Knowledge and practice always reflect one another, change does not result from the development of knowledge alone, and there is an important element of continuity even when change appears to be most dramatic. It follows that the historical and cultural diversity of medical theory and practice must not be regarded as indicating that many of the various approaches to and different systems of medicine are necessarily backward and uninformed, but they should be seen instead as an essential and enriching feature in understanding the nature of medicine. Hence there was no sharp break in medical history when scientific medicine became established and before which nothing medical is worth attention. Rather as King suggests the continuity lies in the practical problems addressed: 'In my view our medical heritage, for at least twenty-five hundred years, has shown a continuity, with a substrate that exhibits a remarkable constancy - namely a constancy of problems'.(15)

Another aspect of this is that the changes introduced by scientific medicine have in some respects been less dramatic than commonly portrayed. Much of the procedure and expectations of medical practice remain the same even though science and technology constantly change; and in order to understand the relationship between medical practice and knowledge, the differences between medical and more exact scientific method e.g. that of physics must be borne in mind. This is a matter of degree rather than of kind and Fleck was perhaps the first writer to analyse and describe them systematically.(16) One way of considering these differences is through the notion of open and closed systems in science. Bhaskar defines a closed system 'simply as one in which a constant conjunction of events obtain; i.e. in which an event of type a is invariably accompanied by an event of type b'.(17) But he goes on to claim that if science is to be possible the world must be an open system in which there are no such constraints. However in order to investigate the world 'The experimental sciences have been able, as a result of theoretical endeavour and technical ingenuity, to carve out a chunk of the uncontrolled world and use it as an object of inquiry'.(18)

Two problems now arise though. The first applies to science in general, and is that scientists may forget they are working experimentally with closed systems and that their findings do not bear a direct relationship with an open system, about which there can never be any fixed and complete knowledge. The second concerns the fact that in medicine no experiment involving human subjects can ever be conducted in a truly closed system. The constant conjunction of events necessary for such a system can never be obtained in practice, because people, and to a lesser extent animals, cannot be dealt with in a mechanical way, as may be the case with chemicals in test-tubes for example.

The conclusions to be drawn from this are that even the 'idealised' scientific method using closed systems cannot produce any definitive knowledge about the world, and that medical method is even more inexact. The knowledge derived from medical research must therefore be regarded as having an approximate and provisional quality and hence be treated with the utmost caution. Whilst the aim behind the development of medical theory and knowledge, in terms of the construction of models containing categories such as disease is understandable as a means of attempting to devise closed systems, the process is especially problematic in medicine. The necessarily selective abstractions required can provide only a partial and impermanent view of the world. Fleck saw this clearly:

> The object of medical thinking - illness - is not an enduring state, but a process which changes continually, and which has its temporal genesis, its course and decline. This scientific illusion, this fiction, this individual entity created by abstraction based on statistics and intuition, the entity called the disease which is virtually irrational, elusive and undefinable univocally, becomes a substantial unit only when grasped temporally.(19)

It seems that we can understand open systems only through our attempts at closure, but such attempts must always be imperfect, and we are constantly tempted to misinterpret and go beyond what the findings gained will bear. Even to talk of reality or truth in any simple way is problematic, as it may leave the impression that access to complete knowledge is theoretically possible. So the exact nature of an open system, except as a conceptual device, must also be cast in doubt.

Medical knowledge (even when considered solely in its biological dimension) is therefore perhaps best described in terms of a patterned construct which is ever-changing and never complete, although some of its features are clearer and remain for longer than others. King suggests that:

> We must firmly reject the concept that any single pattern (or event) has a simple and unequivocal relation to any other. There are always alternatives, depending on what I call the edges or streamers. Patterns, combining perception and inference, have both a core and a periphery. The core may be more or less precise, but the periphery is always vague, extending with diminished clarity to connect with other events.(20)

Even the core of the pattern is a construct and has no final shape. The only thing that always remains constant is the overall idea of there being such a medical pattern or constellation of events. The kaleidoscopic pattern itself cannot be resolved because of '... the eternal paradox that while all things are related, yet we must act as if they were isolated' and hence 'In "reality" there is a continuous merging, but for discourse or for practical activity we break that continuity'.(21)

Hence it is impossible ever fully to discern the whole or to grasp its meaning, and therefore medical knowledge is ultimately indeterminate and mysterious in the sense suggested in chapter one.

The greater part of these arguments can be applied to scientific knowledge and method in general, so that it is not that medical knowledge and method are completely different, only that they have some special features which give an extra dimension to the problems described. The exact status of all scientific knowledge is uncertain, but the humanistic dimension of medical knowledge imbues it with a greater uncertainty, which heightens the difficulty of how practical action can be derived from the insecurity of less than determinate knowledge. The practical and humanistic dimensions determine that medical knowledge can never be adequately characterised as simply a part of scientific knowledge. It is the interplay between the two facets of medicine, the imperative need to engage in practice and the unavoidable insecurity of knowledge and method, that constitutes its essence; and it is only by grasping this that an adequate representation of both medical knowledge and practice can be achieved.

To gain a better understanding of how this applies to knowledge of medical conditions two examples will be considered in the next chapter, schizophrenia and coronary heart disease (CHD). They have been selected because they have come to occupy an important place in our understanding of medical knowledge, theory and practice over the past century, in relation to mental and physical disease respectively.

6 The nature and justification of medical theory and knowledge - two examples: schizophrenia and coronary heart disease

I n this chapter two medical conditions, schizophrenia and coronary heart disease (CHD), will be considered in some depth. The purpose will be to analyse the way in which they have been conceptualised, in an attempt to correct and clarify our understanding of the basis from which they have been derived. This will then be developed into a more general evaluation of our ideas and beliefs about medical theory and knowledge relating to both physical and mental illness.

Many of the most serious medical conditions in the west today have been known since ancient times. They would not of course have been described in quite the same way as they are now or with the precision that is possible with modern technology, but a stable pattern of symptoms and signs providing a line of continuity is clearly recognisable. This applies to pulmonary tuberculosis, cancer and depression for example. However two of the conditions which have been most significant in the present century, both in terms of their seriousness and their frequency, were not described or named until the last one hundred years. These are schizophrenia and CHD. Many other conditions have also been described only in modern times, but schizophrenia and CHD will be focused on both because they are representative of the process of disease classification and because they have played an important role in our current interpretation of mental and physical illness respectively.

These two conditions will therefore be analysed as a way of attempting to understand whether knowledge of 'new' diseases involves the description of a naturally occurring state, or alternatively is a social construct, or represents some other process which has not yet been clearly delineated. Schizophrenia will be considered first because the idea of conceptualising mental illness in different ways is relatively familiar through the arguments developed by the anti-psychiatry movement in the 1960s. Similar arguments have not been strongly and consistently made in relation to CHD, and hence it will be considered second.

65

Schizophrenia

The term psychosis was first used in 1845 to refer to a defect of judgement, in contrast with neurosis which at that time referred to disordered nervous functioning. Later a distinction was made between organic and functional psychosis (with and without detectable cerebral pathology respectively) and between 1860 and 1920 there was an intensive search for syndromes relating to the new concept of functional psychosis. (1) Schizophrenia then emerged at the end of this period as one of the major functional psychoses that continue to be recognised today, and has had a substantial influence in shaping our ideas of mental illness and psychiatric practice in the twentieth century. Many regard it as the clearest example of serious mental illness, so that challenges to the conventional view of schizophrenia have implications for mental illness as a whole.

Traditionally the history of schizophrenia begins with Emil Kraepelin who first described what he thought to be a new medical condition which he termed 'dementia praecox'. His work on this was originally published in 1893 as a short presentation in the 4th edition of his famous textbook *Psychiatrica*.(2) However by the final edition which appeared in 1913 the condition occupied over 300 pages, and by then Kraepelin had proposed three interrelated approaches to the description of dementia praecox; prognostic, symptomatic and aetiological.(3) This demonstrated the growth in significance it had been accorded over this twenty year period. In the meanwhile though, Bleuler had introduced Freudian theory to his understanding of the condition suggesting that its distinguishing feature was the breaking of associative threads, and proposed in 1911 that schizophrenia was a more appropriate designation then dementia praecox.(4) The term schizophrenia soon became established and has been firmly embedded in psychiatric theory and practice ever since.

The conceptualisation of schizophrenia as a disease entity then has had a brief but dramatic history and raises a number of questions in relation to medical knowledge which will be considered here. - What sort of new knowledge does schizophrenia represent? Why has it gained such prominence in so short a time? Why does it continue to be so widely accepted?

There is a wide disparity in the answers given to these questions reflecting an equally wide variety of different perspectives. These will be considered under three broad headings which illustrate the range of different types of arguments used, and will be described in terms of traditional, modified and radical approaches.

The traditional approach

The basis of the traditional approach is the unifactorial disease model described in chapter four in relation to the work of Koch on infectious diseases. By analogy

Kraepelin transferred the elements of this model in their relationship with physical disease to mental disease in determining the existence of dementia praecox. This was most important in his understanding that there was some physical process, which although unknown was nevertheless the essential cause of the condition. Following from this the idea that there must be a single physical cause for schizophrenia has been carried through to the present in the continuing search for different types of biological cause, perhaps most notably in relation to genetics. Many researchers also believe that the basis for understanding the pathology of the disease has already been defined. A recent editorial stated that:

> Neuroscientific inquiry into the most devastating of mental illness is, then, bearing hard won fruit. Few would now dispute that a substantial proportion of patients with schizophrenia do indeed have consistent structural and physiological brain abnormalities.(5)

In this simple and well-defined model schizophrenia is viewed as being similar to physical disease, a naturally-occurring entity, which has exact clinical, pathological and aetiological characteristics. The ultimate determining factor though is the single cause which is potentially discoverable by research. From this perspective the question whether schizophrenia was a new condition discovered by Kraepelin and Bleuler can be answered in one of two ways. Either it could have existed previously but remained unknown until it was properly described and defined, or a new causal factor arose which led to a new disease coming into existence which was first recognised by Kraepelin and Bleuler. What is not questioned is whether there were any social features of the period 1890-1920 which may have been relevant to the definition and enthroning of this important new disease condition. Hence the reasons why schizophrenia came to prominence so rapidly and continues to be accepted are taken as unproblematic. They are simply seen as a straightforward reflection of the existence and prevalence of the condition once it has been scientifically investigated.

The modified approach

The modified approach is less easy to describe than the traditional one because it emerged only slowly as a series of responses to problems identified with the traditional model and includes a range of models within the overall category. However the term modified model will be used in general to equate with the description of the multifactorial biopsychosocial model outlined in chapter four. The first step in the direction of a modified model could be viewed as the introduction by Bleuler of the term schizophrenia as an alternative to dementia praecox. It might seem that Bleuler had significantly changed the focus from that of dementia praecox in his description of schizophrenia, through claiming that some symptoms were of psychogenic origin. However he appears only to have added to Kraepelin's notion of an underlying biological aetiology rather than made any attempt to replace it. So although Bleuler had introduced a psychological component to the model, its basic structure remained as before. Hence Bleuler continued to be committed to the traditional model, but what he had done was to point in the direction of troublesome questions concerning causation, and over subsequent years these have been developed from a number of directions. Some of the more important of them have been as follows:

(1) can the cause of the condition be envisaged in psychological, or psycho-social terms?
(2) if (1) is accepted, does there not have to be a link between the psychological/social causation and a physical expression of the condition, which leads necessarily to the notion of a complex biopsychosocial causation?

These questions about the nature of causation in schizophrenia, have also been paralleled by other concerns about the clinical syndrome. Recently the suggestion has been made that what Kraepelin first described was the clinical condition now recognised as encephalitis lethargica, which has a well-established physical cause and pathology. It is then claimed that there was a subsequent shift in the centre of interest leading to the recognition of the condition which is now described as schizophrenia.[6] However although this challenges the historical account it need not call into question the presently accepted clinical basis of schizophrenia, only who discovered it and when. Of greater concern is the apparent failure of the notion of schizophrenia as it has been developed to embody any fixed set of symptoms and signs, so that there is a lack of unity to the condition. Originally this did not present as an issue because no careful comparisons were made of the characteristics of patients described as schizophrenic, but in recent years systematic studies have shown just how the term has been applied, and though the interpretation of them has been disputed, there appears to be a lack of clearcut evidence of any necessary and sufficient conditions which would form a stable core of symptoms and signs as are required in the determination of a syndrome.[7]

What is left then if the problems raised by both the clinical and causal elements are taken together is a diffuse range of clinical characteristics with no clearcut causal understanding, which would delineate the boundaries of the condition. Yet many of those who fully recognise these difficulties interpret them as containable within a contemporary modification of the traditional model. For example Birchwood *et al.* state 'In our view schizophrenia is best viewed as a hypothetical heuristic concept whose validity should stand or fall by the strength of the aetiological and therapeutic implications it embodies'.[8] They go on to propose '...

genuine integration of medical, social and psychological approaches and the adoption of a broad interactional model as a guide for research and clinical practice'.(9) Interestingly these authors appear to dismiss the need to identify a coherent clinical syndrome, and largely ignore the theoretical difficulties of how to interpret the integration of medical, psychological and social causes on which the model rests. This general stance is not untypical though. What it seems to represent is a determination to continue viewing schizophrenia as a disease entity, whilst accommodating different insights as far as possible within this overall constraint. So the answers that would be provided to the questions about the status of medical knowledge in relation to schizophrenia are the same as for the traditional model, because although the configuration of the disease model is less clear, it is still represented as a specific entity.

The modified model can therefore be seen as a pragmatic device, which takes theoretical integrity and precision to be of less importance then practical utility. Such pragmatism can then be viewed in two entirely different ways, either as an appropriate and commonsense response to the complex and untidy arena of mental illness, or as a stubborn unwillingness to recognise that modifying the traditional model will never satisfactorily encompass the problematic issues raised by the accepted historical determination and description of the condition. It is then from this latter perspective that the need for more radical approaches has been identified.

The radical approach

During the 1960s and 1970s the status of mental illness and of psychiatry as part of medicine were called into question. Nothing about the traditional or modified models was taken to be sacrosanct and schizophrenia which had by then long been seen as central to psychiatry was often made the focus of attack. These criticisms can be seen in retrospect to have come from two main directions; first from an originally unconnected group of 'psychiatric dissidents' who laid seige to the various assumptions of the previously accepted models, and soon became known collectively as the anti-psychiatrists; and second from a group of academic sociologists and social historians who began for the first time to take seriously the analysis of mental illness as a social rather than a physical phenomenon. The present purpose is not to describe this work comprehensively or in detail, but to indicate some of its main directions and further relevant work which has followed in its wake. The most radical approaches which seek to debunk and dismiss the concept of mental illness altogether all involve the notion of *social construction* in opposition to any model which might be interpreted as medical, whilst the (arguably) less radical approaches despite starting with similar fundamental criticisms, propose some new method of *reconstruction*.

Social construction Three types of argument will be explored under this heading; the medicalisation of madness, the labelling of deviant behaviour, and the myth of mental illness.

The idea of the medicalisation of madness arose from the work of a number of sociologists and social historians, who searched in vain for technical criteria which would adequately form the basis of mental illness. Finding none that satisfied them they concluded that mental illness is instead a social construct which has been created and sustained by psychiatrists, being either willingly endorsed by the public or used as a form of professional dominance and control. Pilgrim exemplifies this position:

> From the middle of the nineteenth century, psychiatrists have claimed a special knowledge about madness without providing, to this day, a single shred of evidence to support the assertion that 'insanity is purely a disease of the brain'. Concepts clearly do not survive only because of their logical coherence or empirical validation. In the case of the schizophrenia concept, crude professional assertion assures its validity.(10)

Goffman is the most famous author to be associated with the labelling theory of deviance as it relates to mental illness, and he developed arguments relating to both the weaker and stronger versions of the theory. In *Asylums* he makes the weaker claim that patients who are already mentally ill develop bizarre institutionalised behaviour in response to expectations of them within asylums.(11) The stronger claim is that it is the identification of deviant behaviour and the process of labelling it which constitutes the mental illness, and this position has been developed most notably by Scheff.(12) From this perspective there is nothing intrinsic about the behaviour itself which determines that it is mental illness, and so mental illnesses are no more than labels, without anything more substantial behind them. It is then from this strong version of labelling theory that mental illness is regarded as a social construct, the weaker version not challenging the traditional or modified models, and requiring only the acceptance of an additional layer of argument.

Szasz is arguably the most radical of the anti-psychiatrists, through his claim that mental illness is a myth and has no real existence.(13) By starting from the premise that physical illness is definable in relation to biological characteristics, and that mental illness has no such foundation, Szasz suggests that mental illness is being used as a metaphor which has become mistaken for reality. Szasz's main concern is that personal autonomy and freedom should not be infringed by psychiatrists for their own purposes or on behalf of society. So for him the designation 'mental illness' is being wrongly applied to people who should be categorised in other ways. He considers that if properly understood they would be classified as physically ill, criminal, or as normal, though in the last case they might consider themselves to have a problem of living. They should then deal with this in whatever way they think fit, but should never be forced into compulsory measures which go against their wishes.

These three strands of radical criticism have one thing in common, that they all depend on the analogy between mental illness and a positivist conception of physical illness, and so are vulnerable to criticisms of it. They all assume that if mental illness cannot be defined in biological terms, then it can be described only in social terms, and that to do so is to take away the reality of mental illness. Under such a sweeping attack as this schizophrenia, like all mental illnesses, is emptied of any conceivable meaning, but other approaches stop short of abandoning the possibility of mental illness, and attempt instead to find different avenues to achieve a reconstruction, in which the idea of some form of medical configuration remains.

Reconstruction The anti-psychiatrist Laing focused his work on schizophrenia, but in *The Divided Self* his criticism of the concept of schizophrenia is not directed at doing away with the idea altogether.(14) Rather his interest is in reinterpreting the meaning of schizophrenic behaviour which he regards as a rational response to intolerable circumstances. Hence he relocates the problem seeing it as residing either within the family (which he describes as schizophrenogenic) or the broader society. So although he has done away with the notion of schizophrenia as a traditional illness, found in an individual and analysable in terms of symptoms and specific causes, he has not dismissed the idea of characteristic schizophrenic behaviour caused by a breakdown of mental health in a more general sense. The locus of the problem is now social rather than individual, and so management of it is not irrelevant but must be differently targeted. This is not therefore a complete negation of schizophrenia, but a reconstruction of it as a socially derived phenomenon. Laing's critique is in many respects as radical as that of Szasz, but his interest is different in that he sought to understand schizophrenia in a new way and so had no thought of denying the existence of the constellation of behaviour described as being characteristic of the condition and understood in terms of an illness.

A more recent suggestion as to how to reconstruct behaviour which has traditionally been related to schizophrenia will now be considered. It has been discussed in some detail by Bentall, and starts from a marshalling of the evidence against there being any determinate set of symptoms or syndrome that could form the basis for the concept of schizophrenia. It is then proposed that any attempt to rescue such a concept should be abandoned, in favour of concentrating attention on individual symptoms:

> … instead of investigating hypothetical *syndromes* psychopathologists could make particular *symptoms* the objects of their enquiries. Although there may

remain problems in defining and detailing symptoms (which will presumably not be nearly as severe as the problems involved in validating syndromes), the virtue of this approach is that it avoids the problem of diagnosis altogether.(15)

Hence the intention is to do away with schizophrenia as an entity, but not with the elements that have been related to it, and so to concentrate on them individually and presumably also give them new meaning. The traditional concept of disease and diagnosis is being dispensed with, but the factual existence of mental symptoms is not being denied. Indeed they are being reconstructed as the new building blocks for understanding mental health problems. This would appear then to destroy schizophrenia by a process of fragmentation, but not to question the reality of the constituent parts which are viewed unproblematically as the subject of mental health work in much the same way as before. Unlike Laing's analysis the locus of the problem and the treatment remain at the level of the individual.

Interim Comments

The main discussion of the issues raised so far and the conclusions to be drawn from them will be left until the end of the chapter when the two examples - schizophrenia and CHD - can be compared and contrasted. However it would seem appropriate at this stage to make certain observations which relate solely to schizophrenia and mental illness.

Although three broad approaches to understanding schizophrenia were identified - traditional, modified and radical - they can be seen to contain a whole range of different models which cover a continuous spectrum. The question that is usually asked is then which of these models, if any, may be regarded as most satisfactory in conceptualising schizophrenia. Put in this way it can be seen that the models at the two extreme ends of that spectrum both contain serious flaws. The traditional medical model which derives from a positivist conception of science, separates facts from values and denies the relevance of values in the definition of schizophrenia. Such a view was shown earlier to be untenable in relation to illness and disease in general and is therefore also unacceptable in the conceptualisation of schizophrenia. It is particularly evident that values cannot be excluded from mental illness because the interpretation of perception and behaviour is central to understanding the meaning of the condition. Without the recognition of abnormal perceptions and behaviour there would be no basis for the notion of mental illness, and the presence or absence of associated physical changes has no bearing on this. Equally the view of those social constructionists who take the argument furthest e.g. in the strong version of labelling theory, is also untenable insofar as it challenges the reality not only of mental illness, but of the category of madness or insanity itself. As every known society recognises such a category, to deny its existence altogether is to make the possibility of comprehension within and between societies meaningless in this area of life (compare this with the discussion about Samuel Butler's book *Erewhon* in chapter four).

The more serious problem arises when attempting to determine which of the other models is to be preferred. What becomes clear is that if facts alone cannot be appealed to there is no straightforward standard to adopt. So the large range of approaches still open to be considered, from different views of the biopsychosocial model to the rejection of schizophrenia as a mental illness, are in general in agreement about the relevant facts, but differ as to their evaluation. Some authors seek a common position by steering a middle course. So for example, Venables suggests that though there may be no unitary concept of schizophrenia which would apply in all cases, nevertheless there is a unifying notion which is useful in practice and should not be dispensed with.(16) But this does not resolve the issue because it provides no grounds, other than a pragmatic usefulness, as to why other approaches should be relinquished, and the question of whether schizophrenia should be considered a real mental illness or not, and therefore be properly viewed as discovered or created, remains open as before.

On the assumption of a unified approach an impasse seems to have been reached and a different perspective is required which questions whether it is appropriate or fruitful to raise the issue in this way. This starts from the uncontentious recognition that following Kraepelin's and Bleuler's early descriptions there emerged within western society a previously unknown process, the designation of people as schizophrenic, and that such people suffer in a way that diminishes their lives , which is interpreted within our society as affecting their health. In retrospect it is possible to raise questions and express beliefs about the nature of the phenomenon so designated, but inherently these are not entirely resolvable, because they depend on a variety of evaluations which are not reconcilable. So doubt and uncertainty inevitably surround the concept of schizophrenia and will always continue to do so. What cannot be doubted though is the emergence of a problem which has involved great personal anguish and the disruption of lives for large numbers of people in western society, and in response to which some form of help and care is required in both individual and social terms. Doubts regarding how to conceptualise schizophrenia must not become excuses for a lack of such response, even though whatever is done will always remain open to question.

The emergence of such a problem and the matching response is not then appropriately described in terms of either discovery or creation. We must continue to grapple with these issues on both the conceptual and practical levels, in the hope of improving our conceptualisation and understanding and finding better paths in practice, but not of reaching any final epistemological answers.

Coronary Heart Disease

Coronary Heart Disease (CHD) has recently been defined as 'a condition where the heart muscle (myocardium) receives insufficient oxygen because the coronary arteries fail to maintain a sufficient supply of blood'.(17) Standard histories of CHD draw attention to a number of great men who are seen retrospectively as having defined the landmarks in the process of recognition of the condition. Leibowitz selects three who he considers to be of particular significance - Heberden, Weigert and Herrick.(18)

In 1772 Heberden published the first description of a clinical syndrome which is clearly recognisable as the condition that is currently described as angina pectoris. A century later, in 1880, Weigert described the pathological changes of myocardial infarction following from a coronary thrombosis. Then in two papers, one by Obrastzow and Straschesko in 1910, and the other more famous one by Herrick in 1912, the clinical distinction between myocardial infarction and angina pectoris first began to be made clear, and so the full picture of a 'new' disease entity, CHD, was born. During the 1920s and 1930s CHD became recognised increasingly in clinical practice as a serious condition which was frequently fatal, and in the postwar period it has been described as a modern epidemic, being classified as the commonest cause of death in most western countries.

As already indicated the traditional understanding of all physical diseases has not been vigorously challenged, and this includes CHD. Hence the kind of historical stance taken above fits in with this by taking the presently accepted disease model for granted. A more detailed description of how CHD has been conceptualised will then be given first to show how a modified approach was adopted from the beginning, and the possibility of a more radical approach will be outlined second, although this has not been clearly articulated in theory or in practice.

The traditional approach

The unifactorial disease model as delineated by Koch in relation to infectious diseases has never been seen as adequate for CHD since its emergence early this century, so a modified model has been accepted from the beginning. There are two problems though in conceptualising CHD in this manner. First the primary pathological focus of the condition is unclear and may be raised in three contrasting ways: as a condition of the heart muscle, or of the coronary arteries, or of the blood supplying the heart. It may be argued that these are different aspects of a disease process, but nevertheless they depart from the sharp outline that Koch saw his ideal model as possessing. This indeterminacy in the identification of the pathological lesion has also been mirrored in the conception of the aetiology of the condition. Perhaps because of this uncertainty it seems always to have been accepted that CHD must have a complex multifactorial aetiology, and at the present time the three factors to which most attention are paid are blood cholesterol, smoking and blood pressure. However the relevance of and manner in which these are believed to act is much disputed. For example Marmot describes how there are two main and competing notions concerning cause amongst medical scientists working in this field; those who subscribe to the lipid hypothesis and those who support the thrombosis hypothesis.(19) Briefly the former believe that the principal cause of the disease is the development of coronary atherosclerosis due to high blood lipid levels, whilst the latter believe that it is the formation of thrombi or clots within the coronary arteries. Marmot then goes on to suggest that 'although the two hypotheses are in direct opposition, evidence may be assembled to logically support either view'.(20) It might be thought then that the clinical syndrome is the essential and stable element that is the defining characteristic of the disease; but this is not so. Although some patients experience the classic symptomatology described in the textbooks, many do not, and a minority of patients experience no symptoms and are unaware of having been affected, although it can be shown that they have suffered a myocardial infarction. Such an episode is appropriately described as a 'silent' myocardial infarction.

Thus CHD has always been conceptualised within a modified version of the traditional disease model which has had no fixed clinical syndrome or pattern of symptoms, an uncertain multifactorial causation and in which the seat of the pathology is unclear. This lack of clarity is reflected in the variety of disease terminology which is used, which includes coronary heart disease, coronary artery disease, coronary thrombosis, ischaemic heart disease, myocardial infarction and hyperlipidaemia. The doubtful nature of all the three elements of the disease model might appear to represent sufficient confusion as to cast serious doubt on the customary understanding of the disease and even to its existence as a unitary entity. But this is not the case, and the public perception of the condition as well as that of doctors and medical scientists appears to be untroubled and confident.

The radical approach

To doubt the existence of mental illness was a radical enough step when it was first seriously and cogently proposed in the 1960s, but to doubt the existence of physical disease as a separate entity which is real and identifiable is to strike at the most basic foundation of the modern western view of medical knowledge and hence of the security of doctors and medicine. So it is not surprising that although there is now a considerable body of research which has analysed physical illness and disease as a social construct, this work is not widely known and has made no great impact on medicine either in theory or practice.

Fleck in his research on syphilis was probably the first person to consider medical knowledge of physical disease as a social construction.(21) His pioneering work was first published in German in 1935, but was an isolated contribution which was largely unknown outside Poland until it was published in English in 1979. However by the early 1980s there was sufficient research in this field for Wright and Treacher to be able to edit a collection of articles whose approach they outlined as follows:

> the distinctive theme of the work which we call social constructionist is that it refuses to regard medicine and technical medical knowledge as pre-given entities, separate from all other human activities. Instead, it is argued, medicine is to be seen as a highly specialised domain of social practice and discourse, the limits and contents of which are themselves set up by wider - but not separate - social practices.(22)

They were also at pains to stress that:

> When we argue that medical knowledge is a social product - not some privileged and asocial penetration of the workings of Nature - *we are not* implying that it is somehow unreal or spurious; still less that the activities of doctors are bogus or that disease is imaginary.(23)

Yet it is difficult to see how a social constructionist approach could not fail to be interpreted as undermining the role of doctors *as they have usually understood it*, because it denies the positivistically conceived technical scientific legitimacy that they have claimed for medical knowledge. An extreme expression of how this may be developed was demonstrated by Bloor in his study of adenotonsillectomy, which he saw as having implications for all diseases. He concluded that for each doctor the social construction of any particular disease would be different:

> ... for each general name of a disease entity, symptom or sign present in the corpus of medical knowledge the practitioner must construct for his own practical use representative particular ideas which stand for these general names and which have that degree of particularity which enables their unproblematic application. ... Thus, variation in medical assessments is a natural concomitant of the structure of medical knowledge.(24)

Hence Bloor saw diseases as no more than theoretical constructions, around which each doctor produces his own subjective account of what that disease consists of and how it should be managed. The possible variations are then virtually limitless. From this perspective it would seem that diseases have an abstract and relative quality in practice. Although Bloor does not make the parallel this could lead to a conclusion similar to that of Szasz in relation to mental illness. Then by adding physical illness to mental illness all illness would be viewed as a myth. Such apparently nihilistic inferences make it understandable that this type of study has gained little recognition with either the public or the health care professions, but this should not obscure the importance of such work in providing a counter to the assumptions of the traditional approach. Furthermore the method of social construction does not have to lead to such counter-intuitive conclusions.

Although there is very little research in the social constructionist tradition on CHD, a notable exception is a piece of work by Bartley, who develops her argument in a more positive way.(25) She observes that since the middle of the nineteenth century chronic cardiorespiratory disease appears to have been the major single cause of death in both middle-aged men and women in Britain, but questions whether in the present century there has been only one clearly distinguishable modern epidemic of heart disease as is commonly understood. Through a historical analysis of official statistics she proposes instead that:

> ... we can take as our problem, not the 'epidemic of heart disease', but rather, the failure of the health of men (particularly working-class men) in later working life to improve appreciably in the last forty years.(26)

Thus Bartley does not suggest that there are no grounds for real concern about the state of cardiorespiratory health of the population in the twentieth century, but that there may have been social and ideological reasons for interpreting it in terms of clinical heart disease and of CHD in particular. One example of the sort of process by which this came about is that in 1912 the rules for the designation of death were changed so that causes relating to the heart were given preference to respiratory causes if both appeared on the same certificate, and this seems to have been part of a pattern of events which led to an increasing focus of medical attention on the heart. At the same time CHD became thought of in both the public and the medical imagination as a disease of affluence, and this diverted attention from the failure of overall death rates in middle-aged men to decline during the years of the depression and subsequently. In this sense then CHD was not so much a new disease arising or first coming to notice in the early part of this century, but an expression of a much wider and more general concern about a serious social health problem, which became conceptualised as a specific disease condition.

As with the discussion of schizophrenia the idea of a disease having been either created or discovered is not appropriate, because it would seem instead to have emerged from a particular social and historical context. In one sense the new disease process has a concrete reality, in that individuals suffer and sometimes die from it, but in another sense the understanding of the social process cannot be captured in these terms. What Bartley recognises is that the social perspective will be distorted and misinterpreted as long as the accepted disease model and classification are taken as given. Unlike Bloor she also makes it clear that it is not simply a question of revealing a range of available choices in our understanding of medical knowledge, but that the choices that are actually made must themselves be open to evaluation and judgement, because they have important consequences for health.

The direction now being taken is towards an understanding of medical knowledge of physical disease in terms of both a clinical entity and a social process. One aspect cannot be subordinated to the other and the emphasis of social constructionism is to reveal the nature and importance of the social processes which are frequently misunderstood or ignored. So, for example, as Bartley suggests, 'merely searching for "social factors in coronary heart disease" (or any other disease) may prove to be a self-defeating exercise'(27) because it takes the existence of a physical account of disease as a starting point. However it is equally misguided to subordinate the physical aspect of the process to the social. Each of them forms part of a truly integrated and dynamic relationship the pattern of which can never reach a point where it is finally fixed. This may then help to explain why once a 'new condition' such as CHD has been identified it sometimes continues to gain credibility and acceptance. The social process which was conducive to its original designation would be contingent upon a particular physical pattern which then becomes reinforced and adapted in such a way as to feed back into the developing social understanding. Therefore the social and physical aspects move forward together in a complex interrelationship, the direction of which is not entirely predictable, and with adjustments being constantly made. Often this leads to a relatively stable position where the accepted conception of the disease condition persists over many centuries and comes to be taken for granted. But the emergence of 'new conditions', as well as the transience and disappearance of other conditions, suggests that there is no reason to believe that there is an inevitable permanency about any medical condition.

In describing this more complex notion of physical disease as both a clinical and social process, the danger is of viewing the patient as no more than the locus where biological, psychological and social forces interact. However the purpose of this analysis has not been to detract from the patient and his particularities, but to demonstrate that any simple model of physical disease is inadequate and even the most complex model cannot fully represent the situation. Different perspectives bring different insights some of which may be complementary, although others are not. So any attempt to pursue a complete description and understanding is a delusion.

Final comments and conclusions

During the second world war the medical department of the U.S. Navy established a new diagnosis - 'No Disease: Temperamental Unsuitability' - which was applied to personnel who were regarded as functionally ineffective as far as military service was concerned, and which enabled them to be discharged.(28) From one view this could be seen as not a diagnosis of a proper medical disease at all, just a clever device to enable the U.S. Navy to resolve a publicly sensitive situation. Alternatively though it could be seen as a recognition that the determination of a medical diagnosis does not require the demonstration of disease in scientific technical terms. Ultimately it is a social evaluation of the facts that will count, and the medical department of the U.S. Navy made such an evaluation in designating 'No Disease: Temperamental Unsuitability' as a new diagnosis. Such a categorisation is bound to be controversial because to admit openly that no disease (as conventionally understood) can be an accepted diagnosis is a strange paradox. It illustrates the dilemma of adopting a normativist position when positivism remains the dominant tradition, and begs the question as to which should take precedence.

This example may then appear at first sight as no more than a curiosity, but on reflection it may be seen to be of relevance to schizophrenia. By analogy 'No Disease: Schizophrenia' could be regarded as an equally appropriate diagnosis because there is no scientific/technical account which can be satisfactorily related to. However the argument must be taken further because even if a factual account of schizophrenia were available it would not be sufficient on its own. A process of social evaluation must also be involved to invest the concept with meaning. 'No Disease: Temperamental Unsuitability' is therefore based on a false premise as to what customarily constitutes disease, but within western culture recognising that we can refer to a disease without the certainty of being able to specify it precisely, still leaves a sense of paradox and ambivalence, because of the continuing force of our positivist traditions.

The analysis of this case might then be extended to apply to mental illness in general, but what of physical disease? The example, described earlier, of the designation of hypotension as disease in Germany, suggests that the conceptualisation of physical disease is fundamentally no different from that of mental illness. Once again the relevant facts are open to social evaluation, and it is this interrelationship between facts and values that finally determines their status as disease. Though the debate will continue as to whether hypotension should be considered a disease in *any society*, the appeal to facts alone will not help in its resolution, and the difficulty is that where values are radically different an appeal to them may not resolve the situation either. This is then potentially the case with CHD and physical disease in general. The difference between physical disease and mental illness is therefore one of the degree of agreement concerning values. Most commonly evaluation of what facts are to be considered significant shows less variation, and the way they are regarded is more consistent in physical disease than mental illness. In fact the tendency to use the term disease in relation to a physical condition, and illness in relation to a mental condition demonstrates this point, illness being a term signifying an expectation of different valuations. So there is an ultimate indeterminacy in the designation of all medical conditions whether physical or mental, but it will tend to be greater in practice for mental conditions.

The designation of illness and disease can therefore be seen as providing a necessary structure without which understanding of health as well as the practice of medicine would be impossible, but it does not follow from this that what we call illness and disease have any ultimate and determinate reality which can be described and known. It also follows that to seek 'true' knowledge of a disease at any point in time in any particular culture is a hopeless and misguided task. There are more plausible ways of conceptualising and understanding illness and disease which must be constantly sought, but there is no holy grail through which medicine's quest could ever be ended.

A number of conclusions can now be drawn from this analysis of the process of illness and disease designation.

(1) Facts and values are inextricably bound together in the process of conceptualisation of illness and disease. This is not only because the facts are always open to different evaluations, but also because values also play a role in determining which facts are selected as significant.

(2) Criticisms are sometimes made that the designation of illness and disease is improper because it involves social and/or professional control. Taken as a general accusation this is false, because once it is accepted that a social process is integral to the conceptualisation of disease, social influence and hence some form of control must follow. Therefore the appropriate question is not whether social and professional control is involved, but how it is exerted and by whom.

(3) Many studies have been aimed at determining whether particular diseases are universal across cultures, and a great deal of research has been carried out in this respect on schizophrenia.(29) It may now be seen that seeking exact answers to such questions is misguided, because it assumes a certain uniformity about medical knowledge which is not attainable. This is not to imply that no comparison is possible, but it does raise the question as to the appropriate basis from which to begin. Of particular concern is the common assumption of starting with a definition of schizophrenia which has been derived from the west, and attempting to analyse whether mental health problems in other societies which have different cultural meanings conform to a similar pattern.

(4) It is not just a coincidence that both schizophrenia and CHD emerged at the beginning of this century. During the second half of the nineteenth century medicine underwent a profound change, which involved a new metaphysical

interpretation of disease. In some senses to even speak of disease before and after this period is to refer to different ideas. What the new era both enabled and encouraged was a search for specific individualised disease entities, which were removed from their personal and social context, so it is hardly surprising that many such diseases were described in the ensuing years. What is perhaps less easy to explain is why some such as schizophrenia and CHD flourished whilst others withered or died altogether. One example of the latter is status thymicolymphaticus which was first described in 1889 and disappeared from use after a special committee of investigation pronounced in 1931 that on pathological grounds it had no real existence.(30)

However, a lack of factual evidence is not sufficient grounds for rejecting a disease. The question might then be turned round to consider instead what is required to sustain a disease. This was touched on briefly in relation to CHD but there can be no easy or complete answer. One approach may be to view schizophrenia and CHD as symbolic metaphors reflecting deeply held and shared feelings about modern western society.(31) These two conditions have come to be described in common parlance as a 'split personality' and a 'heart attack' respectively, both graphic expressions of assaults on the integrity of individuals, one on the mind and the other the body. This awareness may then connect with the new metaphysical representation of discrete individual diseases and where it harmonises with them promote and sustain their acceptance and use.

What this detailed consideration of schizophrenia and CHD has revealed is that medical theory is not amenable to characterisation by any unitary scheme. This is equally true of medical knowledge which is both complex and open to contest. Therefore to seek determinate answers to questions about the status of medical theory and knowledge is misguided, and whatever position is taken will be coloured by a particular set of values relating to a particular culture and time. What all societies recognise though is a category relating to health and illness, which may vary to some degree, but retains a universal quality, and so provides a stability to the notion itself. What cannot be said is what in particular must necessarily be included within this category. We can only make claims as to what we believe should be included, which although they may be strong, always remain open to the possibility of revision. Hence to suggest that there is any exact solution to what constitutes a medical condition is a mistake. What medical theory and knowledge comprise are not to be understood in these terms, but have instead an elusive quality such that the limits to medicine and health care cannot be determined with precision. It is this elusiveness which derives from its intersubjectivity which lies at the heart of medicine and gives it its mysterious nature in both theory and practice. The succeeding chapters will therefore explore the relationship between the theoretical ideas which have been dealt with here and a range of more practical health care issues.

7 The nature of medical practice and decision-making

The preceding chapters were concerned with an analysis of medical theory and the conceptualisation of medical knowledge. This chapter will examine the nature of medical practice and the process of medical decision-making to determine how it relates to medical theory and especially whether accepted medical theories coincide with the way in which medicine is practised.

According to the traditional medical model the central task of medical practice is the diagnosis of disease. Hence the exercise of clinical decision-making and judgement is seen above all to involve the ordered procedures of history taking, clinical examination and special investigation carried out in a structured sequence that will lead by means of logical accumulation of data and analysis to the correct diagnosis. This three-stage step-by-step process envisages first the collection and sifting of information from the patient, then a search for and screening of relevant bodily information which can be obtained first by examination and then by appropriate special investigations. The diagnosis should then become apparent from an evaluation and integration of all the collected data. This detailed specification is seen as providing the basis for how good practice should operate and is the foundation on which medical students are taught in their clinical years.(1) However it both ignores and distorts the general pattern of medical work, and further does not provide even an adequate description of practice for that part of medicine (acute hospital practice) to which it is seen to be most appropriate.

The traditional account of medical decision-making outlined above focuses on acute rather than chronic medical conditions and on hospital medicine rather than primary care. In doing so it detracts from medical work carried out with those suffering from chronic conditions, where establishing a diagnosis is only an initial and small part of the whole medical task, with assessment of progress, prognosis and amelioration of the condition being of far greater importance. It also highlights and prioritises the role of the hospital as compared with primary care, although the great majority of all patients never reach hospital but are dealt with solely by their general practitioner. The character of a typical consultation in general practice is very different from that in hospital though. The orientation of the general

83

practitioner contrasts with that of the hospital doctor, his concern being much wider by encompassing a very considerable range of problems that his patient may bring him, and extending over a longer time span as he has an ongoing responsibility for his patients. Therefore precise diagnosis is often not seen as the main purpose of the consultation, and the theoretical model of how clinical decision-making should proceed, as a logical sequence, tends not to be used in practice. Far from the tidy process of diagnosis described above, Stimson and Webb describe a typical general practice consultation as follows:

> Either doctor or patient may interrupt the speech of the other, jump from one topic to another, refer back to statements previously made, or formulate the problem in a different way if either feels the other has not reacted as desired. This makes for what would appear to an observer to be the uneven nature of the exchange in the consultation; there is often a great deal of skipping and back-tracking as the problem is being defined, redefined and reformulated and some kind of solution or compromise is reached.(2)

So the major part of all medical practice does not conform to the textbook definition of medical decision-making. But the problem goes beyond this because even in the acute medicine of hospital practice the more experienced doctors who are recognised as the best clinicians do not follow this model of decision-making either. Characteristically they develop their own procedures and styles which derive from their personal accumulated experience and do not conform to the textbook routines. The root cause of this disjunction arises because there is a fundamental gap between the presently accepted conception of scientific medical knowledge and the experience of the patient and the doctor; or put another way the formulation of medical knowledge has become organised in the past two centuries in such a way as to deny the validity of personal experience. The theoretical process of clinical decision-making has therefore been tailored so as to exclude the relevance of the patient's experience of illness by stripping away those parts which are personal and not seen as belonging to the underlying universalisable disease. The doctor's personal response to the patient's situation has been excluded similarly, except as an additional and subsidiary part of his work, which is not considered to be involved in the diagnosis. In referring to the present century Cassell notes that:

> Only in this era have symptoms come to be seen as purely subjective and signs as objective. Further, the word objective has come to have the connotation of real, in contrast to subjective things which are "only mental" and therefore unreal. This shift in meaning of the word symptom and the derogation of symptoms because of their subjective nature are results of the influence of

scientific[1] ideals on medicine.(3)

The place of personal experience has then been denied in theoretical terms, although it continues to be recognised and even admired when skilfully incorporated in the practice of senior doctors. Hence there is a need to return to a recognition of the place of personal knowledge as has been extensively explored by Polanyi in his book *Personal Knowledge*,(4) and this will be considered in more detail later.

The nature of the gap between medical theory and practice has now been made clearer, but the reason why it should have arisen remains to be explained. Its source would seem to lie partly in the difficulty that both doctors and patients experience in tolerating and dealing with uncertainty in matters of health care. If as suggested previously, there can never be complete certainty about any medical knowledge, then the attempt to provide a detached clinical decision-making procedure which claims to be able to produce such certainty is flawed. Nevertheless in a positivistically oriented culture such a procedure may appear irresistibly attractive because it holds out such a hope. Cassell has suggested five different strategies which doctors adopt to deal with uncertainty, and which help them to preserve their belief about the possibility of medical certainty and the adequacy of the textbook description of decision-making:

(1) De-individualising the patients to make them more like the textbook.
(2) Transforming medical information so that doubt is erased by fiat.
(3) Redefining the patient's problem.
(4) Shrinking the patient's problem to a narrow clinical focus.
(5) Accepting the present uncertainty and believing that it will resolve itself in time.(5)

On the other hand it has already been noted that experienced doctors who are considered to be wise both recognise, at least implicitly, that there is no certain medical knowledge, and in their practice they demonstrate ways of tolerating and handling this uncertainty. However to practice in a less structured and more open way is inherently problematic because it gives rise to a basic tension (as quoted previously in chapter three):

Withdrawal from the patient is rewarded with certainty and punished by sterile inadequate knowledge; movement toward the patient is rewarded with knowledge and punished with uncertainties. The fact remains, however, that to disengage from the patient is to lose the ultimate source of knowledge in

---

[1] In this context 'scientific' refers to a positivist conception of science.

medicine.(6)

Cassell then goes on to conclude that 'To seek certainty itself is ultimately to abandon the patient; to pretend to oneself a nonexistent certainty is to retreat into magic'.(7)

Yet whilst magic as a form of pretence is certainly to be deplored, it would seem that in some other form it is both a desirable and even an essential element of good medical practice. As quoted in chapter one Malinowski wrote of primitive societies in the 1920s that 'The function of magic is to ritualise man's optimism, to enhance his faith in the victory of hope over fear',(8) so dismissing its relevance to developed societies. But the permanent uncertainty which surrounds medical knowledge and practice, as well as the fear and anxiety produced by such uncertainty may determine that developed societies also need certain forms of magic whose practice they entrust to health care practitioners.

The idea of magic commonly raises the spectre of strange and frightening practices, but the notion of magic being referred to here is quite the reverse, having about it a familiar and taken for granted quality, as a normal part of everyday life. Two examples will be described to illustrate this; first the form and content of the typical general practice consultation and second the use of placebos.

In Britain an average surgery consultation in general practice lasts between five and ten minutes. Although many consultations involve only minor complaints which are not of serious concern to the patient and are readily managed by the doctor, others are more serious and of grave concern to both the doctor and patient, but in many cases are still apparently dealt with successfully in a matter of a few minutes. Even more surprisingly patients often claim to be dramatically improved despite the fact that the doctor has reached no firm diagnosis and provided no specific technical treatment or management. The process by which all this is achieved can readily be described but is less easily explained. It has a quality similar to that which occurs in the confessional for example, where some general description of the exchange that is involved can be given, but what is of central significance is unique to each encounter and defies any exact or full explanation.

Before a person reaches a decision to consult the doctor he will frequently have gone through an extended process of lay consultation during which he will begin to form a view about what he may be suffering from, its possible consequences and whether it warrants his visiting the doctor. The consultation with the doctor then represents the culmination of a process of illness behaviour in which there is commonly an acceptance by the patient that some change in the definition and understanding of his condition is to be expected. It is also usually anticipated by the patient that there will be some intervention by the doctor from which benefit will result, and this state of expectation which precedes the consultation is commonly based on belief and trust. There is therefore a preparedness for something dramatic to happen within the short time available, although the appearance may be of a routine or even humdrum interaction between doctor and patient. Typically there are three elements to the consultation process which may overlap and so are not usually clearly demarcated in practice. The first consists of a dialogue between the doctor and patient in which the nature of the patient's problem is discussed and negotiated. The second, which is sometimes omitted and is nearly always very limited in scope, is a physical examination of the patient. The third involves some explanation, advice, reassurance, and prescription of treatment by the doctor. What is clear though is that this is quite unlike the textbook description of clinical decision-making, as revealed in the quotation already given from Stimson and Webb. There is an element of a rational technical process in which the history-taking and physical examination may lead to a conventional diagnosis, but this is overlaid and interpenetrated by the personal qualities brought to the interchange, in which the patient plays an active role and the doctor is much more than a technical decision-maker. The dialogue between doctor and patient is then not only one in which the doctor elicits relevant information from the patient, but of a negotiated interpretation of just how the problem is to be understood. The physical examination, when it is carried out, is often restricted to just one or two simple procedures, such as taking the pulse, measuring the blood pressure or listening to the chest. Although these procedures may sometimes be of value for clinical purposes, their rather frequent and non-selective use cannot be explained solely in these terms. They would seem to have an additional significance: that of a symbolic routine, which may provide benefit to the patient and marks out the special content of the doctor's work over and above that of technical expertise. It allows the possibility of apparently straightforward clinical tasks embodying a personal quality which only gains meaning from the responsiveness of the patient in return, and so is shared by the doctor and patient. Finally the stage of explanation, advice, reassurance and prescription of treatment would seem to suggest that the patient is entirely passive towards the end of the consultation. However this is not the case; first this stage is often not clearcut and patients may continue to relate further problems or other aspects of concern; second patients frequently reinterpret or reject the doctors advice either in whole or in part although they may not confront their doctor over it. This does not necessarily stop them from feeling better though, indeed it may be that for some patients retaining a degree of control over the interpretation of their medical condition and its management independently of the doctor is essential to their improvement.

The patient's personal response is then crucial to a successful consultation, but that of the doctor is equally so. Balint who made a special study of the use of psychotherapy in general practice went so far as to call the emotional and personal response of the doctor to the patient, the prescription of the drug 'doctor'.[9] Far from acting in a uniform manner as a rational technical view of decision-making would dictate, doctors develop different styles of practice and Balint concludes that '... it is not so much the patient's needs but the doctor's individuality that determines the form in which the doctor administers himself'.(10) The power that can be dispensed by such individual behaviour was well understood in the nineteenth century, as shown by a passage from Trollope's novel, *Dr Thorne*. His description of the sinister-sounding but highly respected Dr Fillgrave runs as follows:

> ... the great feature of his face was his mouth. The amount of secret medical knowledge of which he could give assurance by the pressure of those lips was truly wonderful. By his lips, also, he could be most exquisitely courteous, or worse sternly forbidding. And not only could he be either the one or the other, but he could at his will assume any shade of difference between the two, and produce any mixture of sentiment.(11)

That similar references are difficult to find today should not be taken to mean that the personal power of the doctor has necessarily declined, rather that such sources of power are less readily acknowledged and accepted than formerly.

Within the few minutes of the consultation there is the possibility of bringing together the personal concentration of both doctor and patient directed to a particular end. However the chance of successful interaction between them is always uncertain because the ability to communicate meaningfully and understand one another is necessarily limited. Hence the mutual need to transcend this limitation, which applies to both what is produced and how it is brought about, requires an element of magic, of the achievement of something which cannot be readily explained. Balint's description of a psychotherapeutic flash technique(12) could be interpreted in this way, but attempting to analyse magical properties in any structured manner runs the risk of dissipating them by reduction. Although both doctor and patient may be generally aware of what is likely to make for a successful consultation, it is not something they can plan for very precisely or be able to describe in full detail afterwards. Part of what is involved is a striving for new understanding, but part is beyond comprehension and relies on faith and trust, demonstrated by an optimistic attitude from both sides. Therefore a 'good' consultation must involve a degree of magic, and the reasons for it having turned out well must also involve a degree of mystery, and though only considered in relation to the general practice consultation here, similar processes can be observed throughout medical practice. Hence magic and mystery in medicine are not some strange phenomena, but an essential and integral part of medical practice with which we are all familiar even though we are unaccustomed to recognising them explicitly.

There are certain instances though where the question of whether magic is being used in medicine has been raised more openly, and one of these concerns the use of placebos. This will therefore be explored in some detail.(13) The idea of the use of magic is usually taken in western society as something which by definition is suspect and to be deplored, so to refer to placebos as involving magic is automatically to prejudice their status. The root of the problem is that those who decry placebos relate their use solely to a rational technical account of medicine. From this perspective placebos involve deception, first in the prescription of a drug with no beneficial pharmacological component and second in lying to the patient about the nature of the treatment. This has led to demands that the use of placebos be banned, but it is difficult to reconcile such calls with the fact that when doctors prescribe placebos they are frequently highly effective.

One way to attempt getting out of this difficulty is to argue that it depends on a limited view of what is to count as scientific causation as expressed in the traditional medical model, and to propose as an alternative the adoption of a biopsychosocial model, which embodies a more eclectic concept of causation. The effect of placebos would then be acknowledged to be scientific, though the mechanism of their action is psychological and is not fully understood. So this provides the doctor with a scientific rationale for prescribing placebos, but it still leaves the problem of the doctor having to lie to, or deceive the patient and so violate patient autonomy. Hence the view that patient autonomy must require the rejection of placebos is now largely unchallenged.

However it could be suggested that stopping the prescription of placebos is not in fact respectful of patient autonomy as is claimed, but also paternalistic, in that it denies patients the possibility of choosing an effective therapy. A genuine respect for patient autonomy would still seem to require the rejection of lying and deception, but without conceding the need to give up the use of placebos altogether. Patients would then decide whether to accept a placebo rather than doctors giving it. It would seem that neither doctors nor patients could object to such an apparently simple expedient when the essence of placebos is that they contain no active ingredient, so that even if few patients accepted them, there would be no possibility of their causing harm. Yet this apparently logical approach to the resolution of whether to prescribe placebos has not been seriously tried, even though there is some research evidence to suggest that placebos can be effective when their nature is disclosed.(14) Why should this be?

A clue lies in the inclusion of 'humour' in the dictionary definition of placebo.(15) To humour someone may be interpreted in two ways. It may imply that the person being humoured is not being taken seriously and therefore being dismissed, their whim being indulged as the simplest and least troublesome way of dealing with them. Doctors may use placebos in this way to put aside the complaints of patients which they consider to be trivial, or not 'really' medical, or to pretend that an active treatment is being given to patients with diseases where none is available. Such an attitude is clearly unacceptable, but to change it does not necessarily require that doctors abandon medical paternalism, because one of the tenets of paternalism, the requirement to act in the patients' best interests, was previously being ignored. It may then be argued that what is required is not the abandonment of placebos, but a change in attitude of doctors to their patients, which involves them in taking the patients' perception of their complaints more seriously. This is the second way in which humouring someone may be interpreted, one in which the doctor attempts to understand what the patients themselves require in alleviating what they conceive to be wrong. What this does not and cannot encompass though, is patient autonomy. A patient cannot choose to be humoured, humouring can only be bestowed by the doctor on the patient, and for the patient to request it is to negate what it is to humour someone. So if a placebo is correctly described as a method of humouring someone, it would seem that its ethical basis cannot be derived from the principle of patient autonomy, by definition.

Those who wish to see placebos abandoned on the grounds that they are disrespectful of patient autonomy may, however, approach the issue differently by claiming that their use is an illicit means of providing comfort, support and care to the patient. They argue that placebos are bogus in that they merely provide a shortcut to such care, without requiring the doctor to explain the situation to the patient, or to give 'real' comfort and support by talking to him, counselling him or providing whatever else may be necessary. Hence if placebos were given up and replaced with such comfort, support and care, patient autonomy would be genuinely respected, and there would be no need to consider the use of placebos, as any function they might have had would be obsolete. Placebos would therefore simply slip out of use and become redundant. There is much to be said for this line of reasoning. Patients are given full knowledge of the relevant facts, and the doctor is able to provide them with care even though no active treatment is available. It is more satisfactory than anything proposed previously, and yet there remains a flaw in the argument which will be considered through analysing the nature of the placebo effect.

The prescription by a doctor of any and every drug carries with it an extra component that is known as the placebo effect. So it is not possible for a doctor to prescribe only the medically active ingredient of a drug, there will also inevitably be a placebo effect accompanying it. Therefore, those who wish to encourage respect for patient autonomy and see this as requiring the abandonment of the use of placebos, need to pay attention to the placebo effect as well as the placebo per se. Logically this would entail that the doctor explain to all his patients that the drugs they received had two components, part active ingredient and part placebo, and that they should appreciate the existence of the latter and come to a decision as to how to respond to it. The possibility of such a procedure being adopted in practice is non-existent, because it has a ludicrous quality about it, but in posing the question, the nub of the dilemma raised by placebos becomes more sharply exposed. By considering the placebo effect, it is clear that placebos cannot be considered as a marginal issue, but must be seen as central to all medical treatment. The placebo effect reveals that the process of a doctor prescribing a treatment for a patient necessarily entails something symbolic to which the patient is likely to respond positively. It is also not in the nature of such symbolic treatment that it can be requested or refused, because it is an inextricable part of what it is to prescribe a treatment. Therefore, the very notion of offering the patient the choice of accepting or rejecting the placebo effect along with an active treatment, is meaningless. But once the inevitability of the placebo component of all drugs is accepted as something which doctors do not and indeed are unable to fully explain to patients, then there would seem also to be an acceptable place for placebos. Such a recognition would not exclude the need for comfort, support and care by doctors, but would show that they are not interchangeable with placebos or the placebo effect. Rather these different elements form part of a continuum of treatment from the purely symbolic to the technical. However even the most technical treatment contains a symbolic element. Hence those who persist with the arguments for abandoning placebos should also apply them to all medication, and so to propose replacing placebos with comfort,support and care would seem to require replacing all medication similarly. Such a conclusion could hardly be contemplated, even by the most ardent advocate of this position, because besides its disastrous results, it would restrict patient choice and autonomy by preventing the use of active medication.

What is at issue between those who support the use of placebos and those who do not, is not usually whether placebos should ever be prescribed (because even those who are strongly opposed to them e.g. Bok[16] consider them to have some place) but whether they necessarily involve deception. As long ago as 1909 Cabot stated that 'No patient whose language we can speak, whose mind we can approach, needs a placebo',[17] and this is not in dispute. The problem though is that the language and mind of doctor and patient may not always be so readily brought into harmony, or the processes of their communication be made transparent. Certainly every means should be adopted to make them so wherever possible, but with the expectation that this will rarely if ever be completely achievable. Such an awareness limits the use of placebos on the one hand, but recognises their necessary and positive role on the other.

Placebos now begin to appear in a different light, no longer being seen as a deceitful part of a technical treatment, but as therapeutic symbols whose efficacy is determined by the subjective responses of both doctor and patient in each particular circumstance in which they are prescribed. Once a magical element in medicine is acknowledged, placebos no longer appear strange, but can be seen as perhaps the most concrete and powerful testimony to the inevitable place of symbolism in medicine. Placebos have truly magical properties because they are both potent but cannot be explained technically, and they could never be abolished altogether because although the use of placebos per se could be stopped, the placebo effect could not be. The question to be asked is not then whether placebos should be used or not, but given that they have a place in medicine how and when should they be prescribed?

The gap that has been identified between medical theory and practice can now be seen not as simply one between knowledge on the one hand, and the experience of the doctor and patient on the other, but between technical medical knowledge which informs the doctor's perspective and lay knowledge which informs the patient's perspective. The common experience between doctor and patient can never completely close such a gap, as it is an inherent part of their different respective roles. However if this gap cannot be dealt with in some way, the doctor-patient relationship will be impoverished and the healing process impaired. Therefore the task is to find ways of narrowing the gap, whilst acknowledging that attempting to close it altogether is neither a possible nor a desirable goal. Placebos are one means of attempting to deal with this gap, but there are other ways of overcoming the separation in order to produce a 'successful' consultation. These entail a different understanding of knowledge than that of positivism or reductionism; one that accepts a personal dimension as a necessary part of knowledge. Polanyi describes such knowledge as follows: '... the act of knowing includes an appraisal; and this personal coefficient, which shapes all factual knowledge, bridges in doing so the disjunction between subjectivity and objectivity'.(18) Although such knowledge provides no ultimately secure foundation, it allows the possibility of its own transformation into shared knowledge, so enabling the doctor and patient jointly to create and pool their healing resources.

Brody describes the process of constructing such knowledge in terms of a story involving expressive compassion:

> First, the story must appear coherent and relevant to the sufferer himself. It must be comprehensive enough to take into account the suffering experience in its totality, not just particular features of it (hence the inadequacy of medical diagnosis by itself in cases where the suffering is in large part psychological and spiritual). And it must be sufficiently particularised to be recognizable as the sufferer's own story rather than some mass-produced account. But second, the story must help reconnect to the broader society and culture. It must label the experience in ways that indicate how others have shared similar (if not identical) experiences and in ways that help to promote a fellowship among all humans who have suffered. The compassionate presence and participation of the physician symbolizes this two-directional feature of the successful story. On the one hand, the physician attends to the sufferer as a unique person; on the other hand, the physician represents the broader society and culture, the "normal" people, reminding the sufferer that the suffering has not totally cut

him off from the "normal" world.(19)

The tenuousness of such bridges is poignantly expressed by Berger in his story of a country doctor; but it is the willingness to reach out despite the risk of failure which Berger considers to be the hallmark of a good doctor:

> ... he is acknowledged as a good doctor because he meets the deep but unformulated expectation of the sick for a sense of fraternity. He recognizes them. Sometimes he fails - often because he has missed a critical opportunity and the patient's suppressed resentment becomes too hard to break through - but there is about him the constant will of a man trying to recognize.(20)

Such moments of recognition depend on personal stories or knowledge, whose subjective element is both necessary in making the connection, but cannot be fully described or explained. That something significant and positive has happened is certain once it has occurred, but its source remains uncertain and cannot be traced exhaustively. Frequently it is also transient, hence Balint's use of the term 'flash' technique. Doctors and patients can then cultivate a climate where such recognition is more likely to take place, but it is not something that can be predicted or reconstructed once it has passed. So the creation of personal stories and knowledge has a magical element to it expressed most dramatically as 'flashes' or more mundanely as moments of recognition, and these episodes have a mysterious quality because their secrets can never be laid bare in entirety.

These moments of recognition are not isolated phenomena though, but part of a wider process of healing. Recognition is itself not enacted only through speech, but may be linked with the symbolic routines carried out by doctors which have already been described. Such different elements may then be regarded as part of a spectrum of healing processes. Berger illustrates the intimate relationship between the verbal and physical components, so showing that the symbolic and technical aspects of treatment are not readily separable either:

> It is as though when he talks or listens to a patient, he is also touching them with his hands so as to be less likely to be misunderstood: and it is as though, when he is physically examining a patient, they were also conversing.(21)

Placebos and the placebo effect whilst being closely related to this kind of interaction, appear to occupy a special and ambiguous place. On the one hand they may be seen as part of a continuum of symbolic healing procedures, but on the other hand they may be viewed as a technical sleight of hand, representing deception and designed to hide failure. Recognition of both sides of this coin, shows how they encapsulate the opposing forces of healing - positive and negative, or light and dark, - which are invested in doctors.(22) The doctor treads the tightrope between them, and resorting to placebos may be simultaneously an admission of failure, and a positive recognition by the doctor of his own fallibility and limitations, as well as those of his patient and the world which he inhabits. A good doctor will therefore limit his use of placebos whenever he feels able to do so, but when he judges otherwise will make a positive decision to use them in the confident expectation that they will be beneficial. To do anything less is to fail to reach out to his patients, although in the attempt he always risks misjudgment and will sometimes fail to connect altogether. The bridging process is always two-way, and so all the connections which are explored as means to healing, including those of placebos, can only be made insofar as the patient is also responsive.

The skill of the doctor lies in his judgement as to which means of healing to adopt in each case, and the honesty with which he does so. The process involved cannot be exactly specified or assessed, but those doctors who demonstrate such skills are not difficult to recognize. Even the best doctor cannot be successful with all patients, but some will be consistently more successful than others.

The place of placebos is then not so special as might at first appear, because they are part of the acceptable range of treatment that is available to the doctor. However they do highlight the uncertainty which the doctor faces in the prescription of any treatment. This is first because they so clearly unite both physical and symbolic elements, and thus demonstrate that these are not readily divisible. Hence the doctor can never be certain of which of these modes of treatment is operative, or even whether conceptualising them separately makes sense. It might be seen that the symbolic is being made technical, or vice versa. Second placebos reveal the paradox of the frailty and even the failure of the doctor/patient encounter when seen in one light, whilst at the same time demonstrating the force of its healing power when viewed from a different angle. However these are attributes of all treatment to some degree, and the main thing that is remarkable about placebos is that the issues are so clearly focused, because the symbolic and technical elements are so intimately intertwined.

Placebos are not then in a unique position with respect to deception and manipulation. They may of course be used in this way, but so can any treatment. Placebos may also 'work' in a technical sense, even when prescribed in a cynical fashion, but this will involve an abuse of the patient's trust and the doctor's power to heal, such that the foundations of the doctor/patient relationship will have been eroded. Once again though any treatment may be given in a similar manner. Conversely with the best of motives doctors can never ensure that placebos work, but equally the flash technique can never be made to work on every occasion, and even the most powerful of technical treatments may not lead to the theoretically predicted beneficial outcome.

The difficulty with understanding the proper role of placebos and the placebo effect disappears once it is appreciated that to some degree all treatments involve both a technical and symbolic element which are interactive, and that both aspects must always be attended to. In considering the placebo effect Brody puts it as follows:

> So long as medicine makes progress by abstracting only the person's animal features for study, the dominant medical paradigm is bound to view the placebo effect as an anomaly. But the capacity theory of the person implies that no being can be *necessarily* both a biological and a cultural entity without the cultural features influencing the biological ones and vice versa.(23)

The nature of the gap between doctor and patient and the processes of healing described here by which it is transcended, and of which placebos and the placebo effect are a part, has in the main been wrongly characterised and so misunderstood in recent years; and this is what has led so many to take the view that placebos must involve disrespect for patients. There need be no disagreement though that the moral issue is about how doctors should respect their patients. The difficulty arises over what that respect entails, and those who reject placebos do so principally on the basis of a second argument which has become allied with the traditional separation of the biological/technical and cultural/symbolic elements of medicine already referred to. This is the appeal to the supremacy of patient autonomy in the doctor/patient relationship, particularly as expressed in the doctrine of informed consent, and it will therefore be analyzed in some depth.

Until a relatively short while ago it was widely accepted that the relationship between doctor and patient was properly one of medical paternalism, in which doctors made decisions for patients without having to discuss their reasons or seek consent from their patients. The ethical basis for this was usually described as relying on two assumptions. First that the relevant medical knowledge possessed by the doctor was of such a nature and complexity that it could not be adequately explained to patients in a form that they would understand. Second that even if some patients were able to comprehend this medical knowledge it would not usually be in their best interests for them to be given it. Hence it was claimed that the doctor should make judgements on the patient's behalf, not least about whether to communicate medical information to the patient and if so how much. Embodied in these assumptions were two deeply-held convictions - that not all the doctor's knowledge relevant to a particular case could be made available to the patient; and that the doctor should be the judge of how much information to convey and how best to act. One consequence of this was that placebos were considered to be morally acceptable even though they involved the withholding of information, because to do so was seen as a normal and proper part of medical practice. Therefore the negative connotation of the word deception which would be applied

95

to placebos now, would not have been appropriate previously.

In recent times such acceptance of medical paternalism has been vigorously challenged and is now commonly portrayed as ethically unacceptable. It has been replaced by the notion of patient autonomy which underpins the doctrine of informed consent. This requires that patients be given the opportunity to make decisions on their own behalf whenever they are competent to do so, and carries with it two different assumptions. First that given the time and commitment by doctors, competent patients are usually capable of understanding the relevant medical information to enable them to reach valid decisions about their own health care. Second that such information should be made available to them by the doctor. Hence there is usually no place for doctors to judge that relevant medical information should not be passed to the patient, on the grounds that it will not be understood or that it would be better for the patient that he should not receive it.

It is on this basis that the doctrine of informed consent has been described as follows:

> The cornerstone of our approach to informed consent is the belief that the right of patients to participate in making their own medical decisions, usually called the right to autonomy in decision-making, is a moral value worth promoting. When medical care is required, patients should be met by physicians' openness and willingness to present and discuss a variety of options, with the clear understanding that patients can play a role, if they desire, in shaping the ultimate decision. Our instinctive assumption that most patients would endorse this approach was confirmed by a large-scale study sponsored by the President's Commission. Patients do want to know about and have the option of influencing the nature of their medical care.(24)

However there are several problems associated with this, which will be described as of two types, marginal and central.

The marginal problems are of three sorts:

(1) that surveys have shown that in many cases patients find considerable difficulty in fully understanding and recollecting all the information required in making an informed choice. However the proponents of informed consent tend to view this as a difficulty to be overcome rather than a serious limitation of the doctrine, and also stress that it is adequate comprehension and not full understanding or recall that is the appropriate standard;(25)

(2) a particular subset of (1) above arises where the patients' psychological and intellectual poise is seriously disturbed by their medical condition. Carnerie expresses this well:

> Many individuals develop a temporary state of cognitive and emotional

96

impairment after being diagnosed with catastrophic illness. Thus, when crucial decisions about medical treatment are required, they are unable to assimilate information; or worse, the legal need to be informed can rival a psychological desire to not be informed.(26)

The author then goes on to explore ways of overcoming such difficulties and so of keeping the informed consent doctrine intact;
(3) those involving particular types of treatment, which by their nature require the doctor not to be fully open with the patient all the time. An example of this considered by Merskey is the use of psychotherapy to deal with pain and other symptoms.(27) He suggests that the patient must be prepared to trust the therapist if any beneficial treatment is to occur at all, and that this makes fully informed consent impossible. This may then be considered in two ways. Either as requiring only 'ignorant' consent, which is valid as long as the patient has initially been informed of what in general is involved and has given his consent. This is sometimes called a patient waiver. The issue then may be seen not as an acceptable form of paternalism, as suggested by Merskey, but as a particular expression of patient autonomy, in which case it would be only of marginal significance and not be a threat to the doctrine of informed consent.

However the alternative view is that patient waivers cannot be regarded as involving valid consent at all, and in seeking to provide the patient with the necessary information the centrality of the difficulty with informed consent becomes clear:

> Attempting to offer suggestions as to what might happen in any specific fashion would provide an influential hint of expectations from the therapist which the patient might be encouraged to follow. Such a course would subvert the integrity of self-realization through the process of psychotherapy. So, to a greater or lesser degree, the consent has to remain 'ignorant'.(28)

Although this latter interpretation affects the doctrine of informed consent centrally it only has implications for certain areas of practice. This does not apply to some of the findings of the large-scale study sponsored by the President's Commission(29) (referred to by Appelbaum, Lidz and Meisel above) which have relevance for the whole of medicine, and so challenge the doctrine of informed consent both centrally and universally. The evidence from the study that there was a desire by patients in the United States to know about and be able to influence their medical care, has to be set in the context of there being strong reasons which determine that, on the whole, this does not happen in practice. These relate to the effect of the disclosure of information on the patient and to the ability of patients to make use of that information.

... disclosure functions not to produce autonomy as the informed consent doctrine contemplates, but to produce trust that, once it exists, will then permit the doctor to dispense with further explanation.(30)

and:

> Fundamentally, patients feel that they are unequal to the task of making medical decisions, even when provided with information to do so.(31)

Taken together these two comments undermine the doctrine of informed consent, because they indicate that it rests on unsound assumptions. The issue here is less about disclosure of information (because by and large doctors are now more open with patients) than what patients make of that information and how they use it. Jacob suggests that:

> What does seem clear is that the amount of information now required to enable people generally to take courage is greater and that submission is no longer unreasoned: there is now an insistence on making reply and on reasoning why. I would argue that the medical profession has responded to this change. This is not to say that true self-determination has become common: rather it is to say those in authority, in particular, doctors, have recognised that greater degrees of explanation are required in order to secure the patient's confidence.(32)

The suggestion here is not that patients are incapable of understanding the necessary information, but that they do not use it to determine what health care choices are made. It might then appear that doctors continue to enforce a paternalistic authority though in a more sophisticated way; but it can be seen instead as an expectation by patients that a degree of such authority should be exerted by the doctor. Patients do not thereby lose all authority, because of the interactive nature of the doctor/patient relationship, which requires their participation for it to proceed satisfactorily, but they must inevitably relinquish some control in the giving of their trust.

The difficulty of attempting to discuss this in terms of a straightforward opposition between medical paternalism and patient autonomy is that the situation is misrepresented by conceptualising it as that of consumers making simple choices between goals. Three important issues relating to this will be described here. First that there is not a discrete point at which a decision has to be made. The relationship between doctor and patient is one of constant interchange and a process develops through which suggestions about the patient's condition and possible interventions are raised. Second, and following from this, ideas about diagnosis and treatment are interlinked and if the consultation is 'successful' the trust that is engendered will determine that there is a therapeutic strand running throughout it. Therefore a healing process will develop through the context of the consultation, but it cannot be captured by an analysis of the constituent parts alone. Hence it is not typical that the doctor makes a diagnosis, then decides on the treatment options, and finally presents the patient with a complete set of facts as the basis on which to make a decision. Although something close to this may sometimes occur with conditions that are clinically uncomplicated, more commonly the process is far less clearcut especially in general practice as was described earlier. Third, this process combines technical and non-technical elements, of which the most obvious example is the giving of drugs which have a placebo effect and these cannot be disentangled, but the doctrine of informed consent ignores the latter. The question raised by these considerations is not how informed consent can be enforced in medicine, but whether the normal mode of medical practice lends itself to being described in the terms that are required if the doctrine of informed consent is to have meaning.

This should not be taken to imply that openness and truthtelling, as well as patient awareness and involvement in developing their care and treatment jointly with the doctor is not important. Rather that notions of either supporting medical paternalism or patient autonomy as if they were dichotomous and appropriate principles to apply to the whole of medical experiences are mistaken. Also that settling for informed consent as an archetypal and almost reverential expression of patient autonomy, is both oversimplified and misconceived. What they exclude, above all, is the recognition of a symbolic element of medicine which can lead to a sense of partnership and mutuality as an essential feature of the best treatment and care. This non-technical aspect of medicine is not consonant with the debate about paternalism and autonomy. So the attempt to implement informed consent when carried out by the doctor in a formal manner, carries the danger of cutting across and denying the role of trust and optimism as an important part of the therapeutic process. The problem is that the desire to eliminate the authoritarian and dismissive attitudes that are associated with old-style medical paternalism, may also lead to an alternative orthodoxy which in attempting to right these issues is itself intolerant of or blind to other aspects of care which do not conform to the new ideology. Patient autonomy and the doctrine of informed consent depend on an idealised notion of rational doctors and patients to be operated in tandem with technical medical knowledge and precisely structured patterns of health care. Once it is appreciated that medical knowledge and health care provision do not and cannot readily conform to these conceptions, patient autonomy and the doctrine of informed consent have to be reassessed. The role of optimism, trust and magic as non-technical aspects of medicine can then be readmitted and evaluated, and these issues relate to the indeterminacy and mystery inherent in medicine and health care, which will be considered further in different contexts in subsequent chapters.

8 Alternative medicine

T his chapter will be concerned with two issues. First with analysing how the
concept of alternative medicine is understood in western society; and second
with exploring the moral question of how alternative medicine should be regarded.
It will be shown that this second issue will be interpreted very differently according
to whether an orthodox view of western medicine is thought acceptable or not. The
criticisms of the orthodox or conventional medical model which have been
developed in earlier chapters will therefore be applied so as to develop a parallel
critique of alternative medicine.

The first difficulty in considering alternative medicine is that of definition and
terminology.   Currently a number of different terms are used more or less
synonymously - alternative, fringe, marginal, complementary, unconventional,
irregular, non-orthodox, heterodox and traditional. However although these terms
may appear at first sight to be purely descriptive and interchangeable, they are
actually also evaluative. For example the terms fringe and marginal carry a very
different message about status than that conveyed by the term complementary. So
each term implies a different shade of meaning and orientation although relating to
the same subject matter. This plethora of terms is then itself an indication of the
lack of agreement that there is at present about the role and status of alternative
medicine, and makes it impossible to deal with the subject from the assumption of
any common understanding concerning the appropriate attitude to adopt. What then
might the common ground be which could relate all these shades of meaning and
give coherence to the notion of alternative medicine?

One approach is to consider what kinds of medical systems and therapies are
included within the overall term alternative medicine and to try and see what they
share.   There is a very wide range of systems and therapies currently being
practised, and some of those more commonly in use in Britain are:

Chinese traditional medicine and acupuncture
Indian traditional systems of medicine
Faith healing and spiritual healing

Herbalism
Homeopathy
Osteopathy and chiropractic
Creative and sensory therapies, e.g. art therapy and aromatherapy
Hypnotherapy
Manual therapies, e.g. massage and reflexology
Mind/body therapies, e.g. meditation and yoga
Naturopathy
Nutrition therapy
Anthroposophical medicine
Alexander technique

There is clearly very considerable diversity within this list, and although certain useful distinctions can be made e.g. between systems of medicine and medical techniques, and between those of ancient and of comparatively modern origin, this does not provide a universally applicable means of classification which derives from and so pinpoints one feature which characterises alternative medicine.

The only unifying feature would appear to be the negative attribute that alternative medicine is not orthodox medicine. What gives coherence to alternative medical systems and techniques is then no more than that they have all been excluded from orthodox medicine. So there is no necessity or expectation that they should have anything positive in common. What this recognition does though is to refocus attention away from alternative medicine, to the question of the nature of orthodox medicine. If alternative medicine can only be understood by reference to orthodox medicine, then orthodox medicine should logically be the subject of scrutiny first.

Like alternative medicine, orthodox medicine has a number of synonyms - scientific, conventional, western, regular and traditional are all commonly used. The evaluations implied by these different terms are on the whole less disparate than those associated with alternative medicine, mainly reflecting only differences of emphasis. However they can still lead to differences of interpretation, perhaps most notably through the adoption of the term 'traditional' by both alternative and orthodox medicine. When related to alternative medicine, traditional usually refers to ancient systems and techniques of folk origin, e.g. herbalism, but when related to orthodox medicine, traditional refers to that which is widely acceptable to conventional health care professionals. So the same term has quite different connotations in the two situations, and if this is not understood it can lead to considerable confusion.

The more fundamental question though concerns the status of orthodox medicine and the reasons why it has come to be regarded as occupying a specially acceptable position by the state, the medical profession and the majority of the public. A number of important features can be noted which are of relevance to this:

(1) The status of orthodox medicine was not recognised or accepted before about 1800, and it has only received official state recognition since 1858 (through the establishment of the General Medical Council which has as one of its functions the state registration of doctors).

(2) The system and model of medicine embodies a number of elements - a primary focus on disease as a discrete entity, which is an ontological conception associated with Asclepius and viewed in technical and reductionist terms; in aggregate this provides an empirical, testable and hence 'scientific' system; such a system is progressive i.e. has the capability of constant improvement built in.

(3) The model of a professional doctor which follows from this is one which focuses on technical training and qualification and state recognition through registration. The fulfilment and continuation of this role is integral to the medical system because it involves both the definition and the preservation of the medical model in both theory and practice.

As already noted the way in which alternative medicine is conceptualised and how it is regarded will depend on how orthodox medicine is viewed. If the features outlined above in (2) and (3) are thought to be generally acceptable and unproblematic, so that they can be taken for granted as the basis on which medicine should proceed and be developed, then one picture of alternative medicine will necessarily follow. However if the same features are thought to be unacceptable and so problematic, then orthodox medicine will require re-examination, and the role of alternative medicine will also come to be seen differently. These two contrasting positions will therefore be considered in detail.

Wulff is an exponent of the view that orthodox medicine is generally acceptable and unproblematic, and his philosophical defence of this position rests on the proposition that orthodox medicine is above all scientific, whereas alternative medicine is pseudoscientific.[1] In order to make this distinction he relies on Popper's notion that scientists must constantly test their hypotheses in an attempt to falsify them, and in doing so establish their strengths and weaknesses. Only those who are prepared to subject their medical practices to such tests are then to be regarded as scientific themselves and so part of orthodox medicine. As Sullivan observes this reliance on the authority of scientific method '... allowed medicine to go beyond the claim to be the *most successful* medicine to the claim to be the *only valid* medicine'.[2] All the claims of other systems of medicine must then be regarded as bogus, and the designation of alternative medicine as pseudoscientific, suggests that it is not only less successful and so inferior, but that its very existence must be seen as a potential challenge to orthodox medicine and so have no true meaning of its own. By casting alternative medicine in the terminology of science, its rejection is all the more emphatic, and the sole validity of orthodox medicine is reinforced. From this perspective alternative medicine is not just non-rational but irrational and so has no rightful place. Alternative medicine should therefore be gradually eliminated by rational argument and scientific method. Hence there could be no possibility of its complementing orthodox medicine. The fact that the use of alternative medicine is by no means confined to the uneducated and has been growing in popularity in recent years are then inconvenient findings which are difficult for those who adopt this position to accommodate.

Such wholehearted acceptance of orthodox medicine requires that a strict line be maintained between what is considered scientific and pseudoscientific, although it does not exclude the possibility that particular practices on either side of the divide may be shown to have been wrongly categorised and so may be switched. And this is how much of the medical establishment has reacted to the recent increase in interest in alternative medicine, by suggesting that certain techniques e.g. acupuncture, that can be fitted within orthodox medicine's frame of reference and so be subjected to its scientific methods, may be candidates for inclusion within orthodox medicine. However this process does not involve acceptance of alternative medicine in its own right, but a redefinition of certain parts of it. Through this process osteopathy has recently gained state recognition, by the establishment of a statutory training course and examination which are required for registration.(3) However there is a danger for alternative practitioners in their acceptance of such recognition, because they will have effectively been 'captured' by orthodox medicine. They will have been accepted for being experts in certain techniques in which they have specialised, rather than for offering a different philosophy of treatment and care. What is clear is that whilst orthodox medicine is open to accepting different techniques and therapies which can be viewed as equivalent to new subspecialities within its overall framework, different systems of medicine deriving from different theoretical conceptions cannot readily be countenanced or assimilated, because orthodox medicine contains no space for them. The other side of the coin is that techniques and therapies previously thought as properly part of orthodox medicine e.g. the non-specific use of vitamin B12 injections can be excluded by improved scientific method, but the underlying tenets of orthodox medicine and so its dominant position are not open to question.

Turning now to the contrasting view, that the fundamental assumptions of orthodox medicine as outlined cannot be taken for granted but are problematic, two quotations will be considered from which to draw out a number of relevant issues. The first taken from Una Maclean's book *Magical Medicine* relates to the model of medical theory and practice:

> ... there is still the underlying assumption that western societies have progressed onwards and upwards out of ignorance, and have reached a condition of complete scientific rationality to which others can meanwhile only

aspire. But is the sickness behaviour of people in modern societies so very different from the seemingly inconsistent mixture of faith and fatalism, optimism and empiricism, which Brazilians, Indians and West Africans display?(4)

This raises the following questions. Has the systematic development of western medicine produced a growing gap between the knowledge and practice of professionals and the ordinary understanding and sickness behaviour of lay people? An American physician, Baron describes the problem as follows:

We seem to have a great deal of difficulty taking seriously any human suffering that cannot be directly related to an anastomotic or pathophysiologic derangement. It is as if this suffering had a value inferior to that associated with "real disease". If anyone doubts this, let him consider our attitude towards such diagnostic entities as irritable bowel syndrome or fibromyalgia or hiatus hernia, each of which represents a disease in search of anatomicopathologic facts. In a sense we seem obliged to remove ourselves from the world of our patients in order to categorize their disease in a technological manner. We cannot hear them while we are listening.(5)

Hence can the progress fostered by the scientific rationale of orthodox medicine be regarded as unequivocally a good and desirable end, or even when considered in relation to peoples' everyday concerns, progress at all? From this perspective an unrealistic expectation of and overreliance on a particular conception of science has provided a superstructure for medicine, which although it has produced a dramatic technical utility, has by the same token denied and so ignored these other concerns, which far from disappearing have been exacerbated by being neglected. How such a serious and pervasive problem is dealt with in practice, is considered by Horobin who provides an insight into the importance of the general practitioner in addressing the issue:

We place the GP in the position of the well-informed citizen who can mediate between the world of science and our own mundane concerns. But we also attribute to him the power to mediate between those same concerns and the hostile forces of disease. He is the weather-god that is not diminished by meteorology.(6)

What this passage brings out is that the GP occupies a special position as an intermediary acting on behalf of the patient, to overcome the gap between professional scientific knowledge and the understanding of the patient; and this process is not just one of translation but also involves a degree of redefinition of the situation. So the task of the GP is not diminished by scientific progress in medicine but enhanced in two ways. First the role of translating the technical language of medicine becomes more necessary and skilled, and second the transformation of abstract scientific knowledge into an engagement with the personal concerns of patients involves a reconstruction of such knowledge in a manner which cannot be reduced to a formula, however complex. What this shows is that the theoretical underpinnings of orthodox medicine are flawed, because they can give no account of these processes. General practice then undermines the theory of orthodox medicine by demonstrating its shortcomings, but paradoxically also shores it up by providing a buffer between ill people and hospital medicine, which enables them to be dealt with in a technical and reductionist manner. And as the terms of medical discourse are those of the hospital model in the main, they continue to be an important influence on the agenda for general practice, from which it cannot escape at present.

The importance and subtlety of the role played by the GP now becomes clear, and is quite contrary to that held by those who espouse a traditional view of orthodox medicine. They tend to regard GPs as either the inferior though necessary cousins of the hospital doctor, or as flawed models of the hospital doctor who need to change their mode of practice in such a way as to conform with hospital medicine. In contrast to this Horobin places the GP centre stage, and so by implication challenges the hospital doctor as the undisputed role model for medicine.

Taken together these points which have been derived from the preceding passages raise some more general issues which are applicable to a critique of orthodox medicine as a whole. To begin with the actual practice of western medicine does not conform to the structure of the orthodox model; and it is not merely that there is a disparity between theory and practice which can be expected to become less with time, but that theory and practice do not appear to be reconcilable. Simply attempting to apply orthodox theory more strictly is therefore futile, and a re-conceptualisation of orthodox medicine is essential. This needs to start from an acceptance that orthodox medicine has no exclusive validity, and that the very aspects of medical practice which have been denied relevance by orthodox theory are of intrinsic importance and can be seen as opening up the possibility of valid alternative medicine. The previous negative evaluation of alternative medicine, as simply that which lies outside orthodox medicine, can thus be re-evaluated to determine what positive and vital elements can be discerned.

A different model of medicine may then be proposed which has the following features, all of which contrast with those of the orthodox model:

(1) Although the model might be described as alternative to orthodox medicine, its general outline can be traced to ancient times and in this sense it predates the orthodox model.

(2) The model embodies a number of central elements - a primary focus on the health and healing of the whole person, with disease conceived as an expression of ill-health. This is a Hygeian notion which, as described in chapter two in the discussion of Dubos' book *Mirage of Health*, does not entail ideas about necessary progress through the reduction of uncertainty which are crucial to the scientific rationale of orthodox medicine. Scientific and technical considerations are therefore secondary.

(3) The model of a professional doctor which follows from this is of a healer, whose most important attributes are charismatic and whose orientation is to personal and social circumstances, as much as technical knowledge, ability and qualification.

It is now possible to draw some general conclusions from this latter view as to orthodox and alternative medicine and the relationship between them. First orthodox and alternative medicine cannot be regarded as sharply divided from one another. The practice of western medicine incorporates at least some part of the Hygeian as well as the Asclepian notions of health, illness and disease, even though this is not always recognised or acknowledged. Conversely the practice of alternative medicine contains elements of the Asclepian as well as the Hygeian model. The goal of achieving a separation between orthodox and alternative medicine (described previously in terms of science and pseudoscience) is then misguided, and it must be recognised that any comprehensive understanding of medicine will necessarily embody some features which derive from both the Asclepian and Hygeian perspectives. Hence orthodox and alternative medicine which are presently described as two distinct systems should more appropriately be regarded as part of a single spectrum, within which there are differences of emphasis, but without any clear lines of demarcation. The question which then arises is what within such a global system should be considered as acceptable and what should be rejected? Or put another way, how should the boundary be redrawn around this new conceptual system of medicine and health care?

Several points relating to this need to be made clear at the outset. The first is that the search for definitive criteria by which to provide a fixed standard for an absolute division between that medicine which should be considered acceptable and unacceptable is misguided. This is the route that orthodox medical theory has followed and it has been shown to be flawed. A much looser boundary whose parameters will themselves always be open to contest and revision would seem more appropriate. And it is of relevance to restate that the practice of western medicine although shaped by orthodox medical theory is very far from conforming to it, so that the boundaries of western medicine already have no precise outline in reality. What is important is that no system of medicine should be seen to be exempt from criticism and revision, together with a recognition that what is regarded as acceptable will be bound to show a degree of variation in different cultures and at different times. Also this is not just a matter of varying technical achievements, but of the deep-rooted conceptual divergences between traditions. Medicine and health care cannot therefore be captured by a single predefined perspective, and a variety of routes to health must be acknowledged with a cluster of associated medical systems, which are nevertheless held together by an overarching frame of reference. What is being sought then is not so much a new system of medicine, as a global context for medicine and health care, the nature of which is such that it is only possible to give some indication as to the outline that this should have. However a number of pointers will be suggested in relation to orthodox and alternative medicine.

First of all once it is accepted that both orthodox and alternative medicine have something positive to offer, then it is clear that insights from all sources need to be applied to best advantage within the revised conceptual scheme as a whole. Equally the entire new health care spectrum which will incorporate elements from both orthodox and alternative medicine must be open to critical evaluation. One of the claims of those who regard alternative medicine as pseudoscience is that it cannot be properly evaluated. However once it is accepted that the methods of evaluation that are appropriate will be different for orthodox and alternative medicine the problem is cast in a different light. The question becomes how to determine what methods and procedures are appropriate for each of them. It is not possible to give any exact answer to this, but the methods already developed by orthodox and alternative medicine will need some re-evaluation, in order that they can be applied to the whole new system. For example practitioners of alternative medicine often claim that empirical investigation distorts the nature of their healing strategies and is therefore misguided and damaging to their reputation. Although this argument may generally carry weight, it is less convincing in relation to particular therapies and procedures which have dramatic and potentially seriously damaging physical consequences. Notable historical examples, from the period before the currently accepted division between orthodox and alternative medicine became established were the widespread use of bloodletting and of drastic purgatives, both of which have now been demonstrated by empirical observation to be detrimental and even life-threatening to patients already weakened by illness. These are extreme examples whose effects are so obvious as not to require sophisticated scientific methods to demonstrate their harmfulness, and yet their acceptance and popularity continued unabated for many centuries. This is then all the more reason why other powerful medicines and techniques should not be exempt from traditional empirical scientific assessments, even though their rationale may not have been derived from orthodox medical theory. Conversely there are aspects of orthodox medicine which cannot be satisfactorily assessed in terms of technical research methodologies alone, and attempts to do so will misrepresent and distort what happens in practice. As this issue will be examined in some detail in a subsequent chapter it will not be considered further at present.

Another possible guide as to what might be considered acceptable in medicine and health care can be gleaned from observing the situation that existed before orthodox medicine became established in its present form in the nineteenth century. The previous division between orthodox and non-orthodox (or acceptable and unacceptable) medicine was very different from that of today. Two types of practitioner that were deemed clearly unacceptable were those classed as 'quacks' because the basis of their practice rested on the sale of remedies for profit, and the 'empirics' who were prepared to advocate new and often untried remedies without reference to any accepted medical theory or tradition. Without wishing to suggest that this view of either of these classes of practitioner should be accepted uncritically as a suitable guide for today, it nevertheless contains some elements of wisdom which remain worthy of attention. With knowledge of the many therapies which have been regarded as beneficial in the past and have later been found to be damaging, a cautious approach to the acceptance of any remedy would seem desirable, and this applies to both orthodox and alternative medicine. So those whose main objective in promoting a treatment is one of personal profit, whether in terms of money or prestige, should rightly be regarded with scepticism. Also those who make extravagant claims for new or untried treatments should be regarded similarly, and the fact that a new treatment conforms to a particular established theoretical system cannot itself be taken as evidence of efficacy. This is because within the new health care spectrum being proposed, internal methods of assessment presently relating to any one medical system will not necessarily be regarded as appropriate. New criteria of assessment will be required involving more professional openness and collaboration, and a greater degree of public and patient involvement in the determination of what is to be regarded as efficacious.

How then would some of these ideas relate to particular alternative therapies and systems of medicine? Homeopathy will be considered as an illustrative example. Homeopathy was devised and developed in the late eighteenth and early nineteenth centuries by a German physician, Hahnemann, in reaction to what he viewed as the inadequate medical theory and often harmful allopathic remedies which were conventionally accepted at that time.[7] His proposal for a new system of medicine based on the idea of the restorative power and ability of self-healing is a Hygeian concept from which three main characteristics were derived[8]:

(i) Diagnosis and prescription are determined by the totality of the patient's symptoms, and so relate differently to each individual.

(ii) The principle of prescription is based on similars, following the maxim that 'like cures like'.

(iii) Prescriptions consist of specially prepared microdoses.

In addition medicines are only accepted within the homeopathic pharmacopoeia after they have been subjected to and found acceptable by testing or 'provings' on healthy volunteers, to ensure their safety.

By applying some of the guides concerning acceptability suggested above homeopathy would seem to stand up well. The practice of homeopathy is well-established and those who practice it do not appear to do so primarily for monetary gain or prestige. It has a long tradition of empirical testing on healthy volunteers to ensure the safety of new remedies and this equates closely with that now used in orthodox medicine. Indeed homeopathy could be regarded as ahead of orthodox medicine in having advocated and adopted such techniques so early on, and it has clearly not rejected technological methodology where it has been seen to be of relevance. In addition the focus on the primacy of safety is a most important feature of homeopathy in making it acceptable. However despite these indications all the evidence given so far only relates to the lack of harm of the remedies that are offered, and nothing has been said about whether homeopathy is positively beneficial.

The first problem that arises in evaluating possible benefits is in interpreting what would count as a benefit, and there are two commonly held and very different views about this. Either homeopathic remedies can be thought to provide a technical benefit parallel to that of orthodox medicine, or they might be thought to provide a non-technical symbolic benefit. In the former case it would seem reasonable to subject homeopathy to clinical trials similar to those applied to orthodox treatments, and this has been attempted by many researchers without at present any definite conclusion in favour or against(9); though such a position would remain open to revision in the light of new evidence, as would be the case with orthodox treatment. In the latter case the methodology of clinical trials would be inappropriate because the notion of a controlled study would have no validity. This is because the idea of a control relies on the elimination of possible benefit arising from a personal and symbolic source, but this is precisely the kind of benefit which is being proposed. So for example if a homeopath was asked to take part in a double-blind controlled trial, where neither he nor the patients knew whether a homeopathic remedy or a placebo had been prescribed in each case, neither party could know whether a specific remedy had been given, and prescriptions could not be tailored to each individual's circumstances. All parties involved may then lose faith in the process as being one of treatment, and regard it as an experiment from which to expect no improvement. The essence of such trials is to eliminate any personal or symbolic element, and it follows that no benefit can be expected from this source, whether the patients are given the agent to be tested or a placebo. On these two views homeopathy can either be seen to have no proven technical benefit (although this does not exclude the possibility of such benefit being demonstrated in future) or for its nature to be misinterpreted by any attempt to subject it to such empirical testing, so leaving the position unclear.

However these are not the only views of how homeopathy might produce benefit, because they both rely on acceptance of orthodox medicine's methodology by considering benefit in either technical or symbolic terms. What is excluded by this is the possibility that these two elements could be interwoven. It is quite conceivable that the benefits of homeopathy rely on the giving of a physical substance, the exact formulation of which has a particular significance in relation to the patient's condition, and which gains symbolic meaning through the context in which it is given. So to attempt to separate and reduce these elements to their components, in order to lay them open for inspection, would be to fracture the structure of the system and in doing so to misjudge the knowledge and healing power that is involved. Sullivan observes that 'Orthodox medicine separates knowing and healing as activities that occur in sequence rather than in concert'.(10) Perhaps this different and more integrated understanding of homeopathy in which knowing and healing are intimately linked, is the most satisfactory and provides an important lesson for understanding alternative medicine generally. This should not be taken to imply that a technical assessment of homeopathy is always unhelpful and unjustified, but that to conceive of it only in technical terms or only in symbolic terms, or even in both technical and symbolic terms but separately, is to give a partial account which is misleading and destructive.

This more complete view raises a new dimension of the problem concerning acceptability though, because the personal responsiveness of the practitioner and the patient and their belief in the benefit of the treatment become the wellspring of its action. So to try to assess its efficacy outside this context is not valid, and this conclusion would seem to apply to all alternative systems of medicine and therapies. Therefore aspects of personal behaviour which are not quantifiable become part of what makes for acceptability, and to search for guidelines beyond the sort of general suggestions that were given earlier would appear to be futile.

The further lesson to be drawn is that this conclusion should be applied to orthodox medicine as well. Technical assessment of orthodox medicine should never be seen as the only relevant form of evaluation, and deciding on its general acceptability will also require a consideration of the personal and symbolic elements which are once again not amenable to exact specification. The fact that trials of treatment are controlled by the use of placebos is testimony to how effective the placebo component of all treatments is. However rather than ignoring this symbolic element of treatment, what is required is a recognition of its role, and other means need to be found to describe and explore it.

So the different systems of orthodox and alternative medicine can both be related to a global context of medicine and health care within which some general guidance as to acceptability can be discerned. However any more precise definition of acceptable boundaries is illusory, because no one system has absolute priority or holds out any genuine prospect of defining all that may be encompassed by medicine and health care. Gaining an understanding of the period before orthodox and alternative medicine were distinguished helps in demonstrating that the creation of such a sharp division between them is based on false assumptions. Orthodox medicine has not and could not attain the unique and separate status which is ascribed to it by its theoretical assumptions. More realistically it has represented the refining and expansion of one pole of medicine, to great technical advantage, but to the detriment of a fuller and more complete view of medicine. The notion of medicine which is alternative is a demonstration of this failure of vision, and the restoration of a more comprehensive conception must involve the reintegration of orthodox and alternative medicine and hence the submergence of their completely separate identities. The insights of orthodox medicine in the modern era will remain largely intact, though humbled and redirected by being placed in a wider context. Alternative medicine will also re-emerge in a new guise, requiring refinement through critical scrutiny; but above all the principles which it embodies will return to centre stage and no longer be demoted to a subsidiary or peripheral position. It is not though that alternative medicine will have triumphed over orthodox medicine, but that they will have both been transformed by a different and more comprehensive conception the detail of which has yet to be determined, but whose roots derive from a reassertion of the ancient understanding of the proper relationship between Hygeia and Asclepius.

9 Medical technology and research

W hen defined in a broad sense technology has always had a place in medicine, as it was involved from the earliest times in the simplest preparation of medicines, as well as ancient procedures varying for example from acupuncture to the trephining of skulls. However during the past two centuries the growth and widespread use of technology throughout all aspects of medicine have produced a new and different relationship. Jonas has described this process in respect of technology in general as follows:

> Now, *techne* in the form of modern technology has turned into an infinite forward-thrust of the race, its most significant enterprise, in whose permanent, self-transcending advance to ever greater things the vocation of man tends to be seen, and whose success of maximal control over things and himself appears as the consummation of his destiny.(1)

Diagnostic investigations, although they represent only a part of medical technology, have had a particularly significant role in this, strongly influencing the genesis and development of modern western medicine. They will therefore form the main subject of the analysis presented here.

Two distinct phases can be discerned in this process. The first was most evident in the nineteenth century when the focus of medical attention changed from the patients' description of their illnesses to the doctors' description of diseases. During this period the increasing use of and reliance on instruments to gain access to and knowledge of diseases viewed as entities, demonstrated the importance of technology in fostering this new perspective. The first use of the stethoscope by Laennec in 1816, and its subsequent general application in practice is perhaps the most powerful symbol of this change. This technical development was more than a new adjunct to medicine, because it had an influence on its development and understanding. When such diagnostic instruments came into routine use, they acted together with the different role being accorded to post-mortems, to transform medical knowledge by emphasising the place of pathological detection and

113

description. This then altered the doctor/patient relationship. The stethoscope gave the doctor more intimate knowledge of the patient's body, and simultaneously distanced him from the patient.

This gap between doctor and patient widened with the advent of more sophisticated instruments, and eventually led to the second phase of development which took place mainly in the twentieth century. It involved the introduction of instruments and tests which do not simply enhance the doctor's own sensory powers, as occurred in the nineteenth century, but add to or take over from them by producing images and readings which became seen as superior substitutes by improving on the subjective detection of signs. A symbolic marker in this shift of perception was the introduction of X-ray examinations by Roentgen in 1895 and the development in the twentieth century of routine X-rays and most notably chest X-rays. Their significance was that they became used for a range of purposes - for patients with lung conditions, for the more general investigation of hospital patients, and later for the screening of whole populations. The chest X-ray came to be regarded as providing 'hard' and therefore essential information about the lungs which could be stored for future reference and comparison. By contrast auscultation with a stethoscope is transitory and appears less accurate and reliable, having a subjective or 'soft' quality which is less dependable. So the doctor became distanced from his own clinical experience as well as from the patient. Reiser concludes from this that:

> Many modern physicians thus seem to order the value of medical evidence in a hierarchy: facts obtained through complex scientific procedures they regard as more accurate and germane to diagnosis than facts they detect with their own senses, which in turn, they value more than facts disclosed by the patient's statement.(2)

Hence with the increasing use of technology 'The word descriptions of the doctor were challenged just as the word descriptions of the patient had been'.(3)

The routine use of testing and screening which now not only involves chest X-rays, but includes ECGs and batches of blood and urine tests as a minimum requirement, has become part of the new orthodoxy. It has become standard to collect and record this level of technical data, failure to do so being tantamount to negligence; and this is only a baseline to which selected specialised investigations must be added. The primacy given to this activity then makes it all too easy for hospital patients to become viewed by doctors as principally a source for the generation of technical data, which can be interpreted without direct reference to them. Therefore the concerns expressed by patients may be ignored, or more commonly be considered as if separate from and subsidiary to the technical evidence.

These worries are often framed in terms of the increasing reliance of medicine on more and more sophisticated and widely applied technology, as if the process could be slowed or reversed without any fundamental change to the medical system. But the problem goes far deeper than this because technology plays a significant part in the present conceptualisation of western medicine. In fact technology has become so bound up with the predominant biomedical model, as to form an integral part of it. How though has technology reached this position, and why have doctors become so dependent on it? First of all it provides the tangible evidence that medicine is properly 'scientific'. This involves an image of equipment, machines and quantification as providing precision and certainty, and so gives the appearance of the doctor being in control. Thus we may encounter the paradox where the patient's condition is deteriorating, but because the focus is on technology which can give an accurate description of complex bodily functions, it may appear that the situation is being successfully dealt with. So the doctor may express surprise when the patient dies, despite the fact that a series of blood results all fall within the normal range. Also it is in the nature of technology that there are invariably possibilities for improvements and new inventions. Consequently new models and applications as well as new equipment and medicines are constantly being developed, and this is of great significance in presenting western medicine as being progressive. It has become the most powerful means by which patients, the public, and health care workers identify medicine with optimism and hope. Patients frequently request tests and technical procedures, and have greater faith in them than they do in their doctors' own judgements. The difficulty for doctors is that because the medical model they accept relies on a rationale which is so heavily dependent on technology, they are in a problematic position in attempting to dissuade patients from becoming similarly dependent. The role of technology is now so embedded in the theory, practice and rhetoric of western medicine, that health care professionals and the public are equally involved in a cycle of reinforcement which is enormously difficult to challenge let alone break. But it is only by directly confronting this issue, that the criticisms made previously of western medicine can be given a more specific and concrete character, and this chapter will be mainly concerned with addressing this topic as well as the related one of how to assess health care and medical technology by research.

The fundamental assumption on which the present status of medical technology and research rests is that medical theory and knowledge are unitary. A major theme of analysis in previous chapters has been that this is flawed, and once this is accepted medical theory and knowledge can always be contested, and so the status of medical technology must also be open to question. Further it follows that the types of researchers, and their associated research methods which are designed to investigate and assess these areas, should reflect this position. Hence an open and undogmatic approach should be adopted in respect of the methodology and the conclusions that may be drawn from research. Unfortunately this is the reverse of what is presently accepted in western medicine and the following analysis attempts to demonstrate why this is so.

One of the features of orthodox medical theory (more fully described in chapter seven and referred to above) is the notion that continuous progress is an inevitable part of western medicine and relies on developments in technology and research. More than anything else such developments are seen to distinguish orthodox medicine as 'scientific' and uniquely valid. Technology and research are then the standard bearers of western medicine, and they reinforce each other in the way they are related. Improvements in technology require research, and research depends on new technology requiring investigation. This is the practical expression of western medicine's reliance on scientific rationalism and empiricism, and it is commonly assumed from this not only that medicine and medical technology are perfectible in theory, but that the appropriate research methodology is as well. In fact it is thought by many that a near-ideal model as to how medical research should proceed has already been devised in the form of the randomised controlled trial (RCT). Cochrane was the founding father of the RCT, and he promoted its use in his famous Rock Carling Fellowship monograph entitled *Effectiveness and Efficiency*,(4) in which he argued that the RCT was not only of use in evaluating clinical treatment but could also be applied in assessing health care policy. It was not that the RCT was thought to be appropriate in all situations, but that it contained features which made it the gold standard in the evaluation of clinical treatment and health care, against which other methods could be measured and compared. So it has come to represent the pinnacle of a hierarchy of methods, giving them a coherence through which they can be viewed as embodying the accepted wisdom of how medical research should be conducted.

The methodological issues involved in medical research are complicated by the fact that such research is usually divided into two rather different activities - clinical research and health services research. Clinical research is mainly concerned with the investigation, diagnosis, causation and management of disease in individuals, whereas the focus of health services research is the distribution of health and disease within populations and delivery of services to them. Now the first problem for those who support the orthodox view that there is a cluster of research methods associated with the paradigm of research standards embodied in the RCT, is that if there is to be unity of method it must be applicable to these two main types of research. The usual way of attempting to deal with this is then to claim that clinical research is purer, more exact and dependable than health services research, and so provides an appropriate model for it.

However this leads to serious differences of interpretation between those working in health services research, especially between epidemiologists (who are usually medically trained) and social scientists. The debate between them commonly focuses on the differences between quantitative and qualitative methodologies, and the divergent assumptions and goals of those who pursue each of them. The following comments selected from an exchange between an epidemiologist who was also Director of a Health Service Research Unit and a sociologist, highlight the differences:

> *Director*: We've got to undertake good, credible scientific research. Science is respected and understood by clinicians (after all it's the foundation of medicine).
>
> *Sociologist*: Do you mean science in general or a particular image of 'hard' science like economics with all its equations. To my mind, what I do as a medical sociologist is just as scientific.
>
> *Director*: You're entitled to your view naturally, but clinicians won't understand what you do. The model of science they know is an experimental one - the randomised controlled trial used to test drugs and surgical procedures. We can test health services in exactly the same way.
>
> *Sociologist* (a later response): I was thinking of ethnography, which means you have to immerse yourself in the situation and talk to the people involved like an anthropologist would. That's just one example of an approach which gets away from counting events and controlling for extraneous variables. It's about trying to understand what is going on, almost through the eyes of the participants themselves.(5)

So the Director in following clinical research methods takes for granted that disease categories and causal variables are given, and that experimental methods which claim to provide universal solutions are appropriate. The sociologist on the other hand concentrates on the processes and meaning involved in health care and seeks for explanations at a social level. Often this does not require an experimental method and is not aimed at providing universal solutions.

What is at issue here is not whether quantitative or qualitative research has exclusive credibility in health services research, but whether one has a superior status, and the Director clearly considers that quantitative research is superior. Without such a recognition it seems that for him there is nothing solid or dependable to relate to, so that qualitative research can be no more than a rather marginal addition to the main research effort. The sociologist on the other hand sees quantitative and qualitative methods as addressing health care issues in different but complementary ways. The crucial contrast between these two approaches is the division between an absolutist and a more plural and open method. Chalmers supports the latter when he states:

> that studies in epidemiology and community health cannot hope to benefit

greatly by conscious application of some generalised notion of "the scientific method", whether the source of that method be philosophical argument or an analysis of physics.(6)

Now the tension between the two approaches is usually seen as being most relevant to health services research, because the subject matter combines an interest in clinical and social matters and hence the different perspectives of clinical and social science. But Chalmers' analysis is of particular interest, because by making the analogy with the research method in physics, the spotlight is turned away from health services research to scientific method in medicine more generally. The question which this raises is whether reliance on one narrow interpretation of 'scientific method' involving experimental quantitative research is appropriate not only for health services research but for clinical research. Thus the debate about research methods needs to be conducted in relation to the whole of medical research, and not be concentrated on health services research. The argument then becomes focused on the orthodox interpretation of medical science and research method and their reliance on positivism, which assumes that they are factually based and separated from considerations of value. It is only by mounting a challenge at this more general level that it is possible to reach a different understanding, which can incorporate other modes of research and place them on an equal footing.

What is flawed in the positivist methodology is not only that it denies the relevance and status of a range of research methods, but that it also falsely claims to produce knowledge which is value-free. Therefore it prevents the possibility of any alternative views being developed, and so has a restricting and conservative influence, as suggested in this passage by Chalmers:

> Insofar as knowledge acquired by way of positivist methodology can lead to no deep understanding of social or other phenomena, it cannot reveal ways in which society can be radically changed. In a very real sense positivism operates in a way that preserves the status quo. Knowledge based on positivist methodology is not value-free, but works in the interest of those who have most to gain from an absence of fundamental change.(7)

It follows from this that continuing to persist with a positivist methodology in medical research has two interrelated effects. First it maintains the status of clinical research scientists and those who work with them as special and superior, through their being seen as upholding the ideals of medical progress. The ideological importance of this position is difficult to exaggerate because it gives them a position of great influence and power within medicine as a whole. The leaders in medicine only retain their credibility by virtue of their research or close association with research, and must conform to the accepted research methods. So the medical hierarchy of hospital doctors, general practitioners and public health doctors is reinforced, because general practice research is often seen as less pure than hospital research by including personal perspectives, and public health research even less sound by incorporating social and political dimensions. Second positivist methodology channels criticism of research method into addressing concerns only at a secondary level. An example of this is the literature regarding the ethics of RCTs, where a great deal of attention is given to such issues as the role of informed consent,(8) but without any more fundamental examination of the basis on which RCTs are thought to be suitable in the first place.

What the questioning of the status of positivist methodology brings out is that no one method or set of methods can produce absolute and definitive knowledge because such knowledge is not available. Thus there is no ideal method or gold standard, and once this is appreciated the RCT assumes a less exalted position. There are some occasions when it will be judged the most appropriate method, but the knowledge derived from such research will never be wholly pure or dependable, and must be critically assessed as with any other method. Chalmers has made the following general observation, but it is equally applicable to medical science and research:

> The common, horrified reaction to the abandonment of the idea of a universal, ahistorical method or set of standards, which sees the move a complete abandonment of rationality, results, I suggest, from a failure to distinguish between the rejection of unchanging, universal method or standards, on the one hand, which I, for one, advocate, and the rejection of all method and standards on the other, which I resist.(9)

Yet all the evidence goes against such a change being widely accepted. It has long been known that medical technology tends to perform less well in practice than is generally claimed, because for example there are problems with the standardisation of instruments, inter-observer error and differences in the interpretation of results. Additionally only a minority of medical procedures and treatments in general use have ever been subjected to research assessment.(10) However neither of these factors has significantly altered the view of both health care professionals and the public that the increasing use of scientific technology allied to medical research as conceptualised in the way described here, is the only conceivable way forward. It is widely recognised that mistakes can be made which have disastrous consequences, e.g. the thalidomide tragedy, but the fact that they are accepted with only a marginal impact on the continuation of the overall process, testifies to the strength of the underlying ideas. So their force can only be understood in terms of a new ideology in which the prevailing use of medical technology and research is the practical expression of power and progress in western medicine. This enables the identification and deployment of the accepted form of medical knowledge and provides the means by which the structure and status of orthodox health care professions are maintained. During the present century this alliance of technology with research has been instrumental in determining both the moral and conceptual framework of western medicine, and it is only through rethinking the relationship that real change will be possible.

It will now be shown why this corpus of research methodology, epitomised by the idealised structure of the RCT is inadequate, because it either focuses attention on a narrow and restricted interpretation of medicine at the expense of a more inclusive and balanced notion, or if applied to a wider medical conception distorts what it attempts to evaluate. Two examples will be given to illustrate this, which represent on the one hand the assessment of a high technology investigation and on the other a more mundane and commonplace medical procedure. They are Computed Tomography (CT) Scanning and the management of high blood pressure respectively.

CT Scanning is a special diagnostic procedure which combines radiological and computer techniques, so in essence it is an extremely sophisticated development of X-rays. There are now two types of machine available, the brain scanner and the whole body scanner. The brain scanner was developed in Britain and the DHSS initially installed a single prototype machine in one hospital in 1971 with the intention that there should be a planned programme of evaluation and development. However this cautious approach was overtaken by events because in 1975 the prototype of a whole body scanner became available and this machine was soon being widely purchased without any such careful planning, a pattern which was followed throughout the world. CT Scanners are both expensive and have dramatic appeal, so that the provision of one soon became a symbol of pride to which every general hospital and its associated community aspired, aided and abetted by the hospital doctors who would take charge of them.

Even if health authorities have clear policy objectives concerning the development of new equipment and services, Stocking(11) suggests that a number of ways may be found to get round them in practice:

(1) There may be routine replacement of equipment, but with the next generation of equipment leading to new activities.

(2) A new service may be introduced by a keen clinician, simply by squeezing others. At the point when the health authority becomes aware of it and feels the need to make a decision there may be a local demand for that service.

(3) New consultants may be appointed with special interests but without that being clear to local managers.

(4) Consultants find other interest groups and perhaps set up local appeals to raise the funds for new technology (this was particularly important in relation

to CT Scanners and appeals for charitable donations became a familiar aspect of life for many hospitals in the 1970s and 1980s).

Those who take a strictly rationalist approach are horrified by such developments, and regard what has happened with CT Scanners as symptomatic of a general relationship which has developed between technology and medicine as a whole, though the results are not usually so visible or dramatic. Thus the scenario which is painted is of technology out of control, with no certainty of benefit and ever-escalating costs. Now the issue to be addressed is not to question this conclusion directly, but the way in which it is usually interpreted by the medical establishment and the solutions that they offer. Jennett is a highly respected representative of this position and has made a substantial study of the benefits and burdens of high technology medicine.(12) He concludes that what is required is a coherent policy involving institutional arrangements for managing technology based on well understood and accepted methods of research, and that this will lead to a more orderly and rational approach. Whilst agreeing about the importance of preventing technology burgeoning uncritically, it will be argued that simply applying a rational programme of evaluation does not deal with the root of the problem, and so is likely to fail. Most importantly no serious consideration is given to the question of why the public and health care professionals alike appear so easily wooed by sensational and unproven techniques.

A clue as to how to make sense of this is contained in the following quotation from Cassell:

> Recovery from suffering often involves borrowing the strength of others as though persons who have lost parts of themselves can be sustained by the personhood of others until their own recovers. This is one of the latent functions of physicians: lending strength.(13)

Now the means of lending strength in medicine is usually through the encouragement of an optimistic outlook, and as already indicated, within western societies the glamour and promise of technology have become an important way of promoting and sustaining that optimism. So technology rather than the personal support of physicians referred to by Cassell has assumed great significance in this process. The problem then is that the development of a traditional evaluation programme necessarily involves a sceptical outlook which will be in tension with this other optimistic aspect of medicine. The customary response to this is to deny that certain features such as optimism make any sense within a rational system, and so they can only be dealt with by attempts at suppression. This is because the research tools of scientific rationalism when confronted with the growth of medical technology, can only engage with it on its own terms. Therefore the possibility of escalating technology being assessed and controlled without medical optimism being displaced is not even considered.

For this to happen the shortcomings of a positivist conception of medical science (as described in chapter four) have to be acknowledged. This is then a prerequisite to recognising first of all that optimism, which depends on the establishment of trust, is of central importance to medicine, and cannot be dismissed as irrational and so be ignored or discouraged. And this argument parallels that relating to the understanding of alternative medicine described in chapter seven. Second it allows the recognition that assessing technology is an imprecise task, because what constitutes benefits and costs is contestable. Consequently how technology is viewed and the place it is accorded within any medical system would be expected to vary. So the acceptance of optimism as an important and integral feature of a medical system, and the way it is understood, will itself play a role in the process of evaluating technology. Thus reconceptualising western medicine so as to include a legitimate place for optimism will both recast the place of technology and allow for a different expression of the role of optimism.

Once the status of technology and the research associated with it have been challenged in this way, highly visible and dramatic techniques such as CT Scanning do not have to be the source through which optimism in medicine is expressed. So there is the prospect of the self-perpetuating cycle of innovatory pressures which leads to constant escalation being erased or broken. In such a different climate assessment could change from being primarily a brake on unrestrained development to that of a more positive guiding role. The need for research would not be lessened but would be reshaped to incorporate an understanding of the values and meanings which people attach to medical techniques and procedures. There has been an overdependence on exclusive medical expertise, and what is required is a redressing of the balance, to enable lay and professional perspectives to attain a more appropriate and sustainable equilibrium. A narrow reliance on rationalist scientific methods of research is clearly counter-productive and a more detailed discussion of this issue follows later in the chapter.

Turning now to the management of high blood pressure, it will be shown that the application of a rationalist technical approach to research can influence such everyday procedures in a way that parallels that described above in relation to high technology. In clinical practice blood pressure in an adult is usually judged against an 'ideal standard' of 120mm Hg systolic and 80mm Hg diastolic (120/80), more attention being given to the diastolic than the systolic pressure. In the postwar period there was a gradual change of emphasis from the earlier unifactorial model of disease to the multifactorial model. This led to a reconceptualisation of high blood pressure from its former status as a distinct pathological entity to that of a risk factor. So where previously only a very small proportion of the adult population had been regarded as hypertensive, much larger numbers came to be included as the new model gained acceptance. A reflection of this was that during the 1970s a number of large-scale trials were conducted to assess the effect of treatment on diastolic pressures of 90-110, which was described as mild to moderate hypertension. The introduction of such terminology was itself significant, the rationale for it being that because raised blood pressure had been shown to be a graded risk factor for cardiovascular disease, levels of blood pressure only slightly above the 'ideal standard' might if reduced lead to an equivalent reduction of risk. Although the change in risk would be slight for each individual, the large numbers of people concerned would combine to produce a significant effect on a population basis. The logic of this argument appears sound when considered on its own terms, but fails to take account of other relevant factors.

First of all the setting up of largescale and well publicised trials tends to have an effect on practice irrespective of the findings. In this case the trend was for doctors to treat people as hypertensive at lower levels of blood pressure than previously before results were available from any of the trials. Although this is difficult to document conclusively it fits in with other changes, notably screening for high blood pressure which was also encouraged at this time, both in multiphasic screening programmes and through opportunistic screening (or case finding) in general practice. So there was not a straightforward progression whereby a new hypothesis about high blood pressure was tested and only implemented if the findings were positive. Rather there was a shift in medical thinking about high blood pressure, and part of the role of carrying out trials was to reflect and confirm the change.

Second the research described takes no account of the way in which the measurement of blood pressure is used in practice, and the effects that changes in its use may have. A typical general practice consultation can be thought of as including two strands, a technical rationalist element of diagnosis and treatment, and a non-technical, personal or symbolic element (see chapter six for a fuller description of this). The latter is of special relevance for the patient in fostering optimism and trust, and there are certain symbolic routines which are carried out fairly frequently by the doctor and help to encourage these attributes. Four of these which are often used are taking the pulse, measuring the temperature, listening to the chest and measuring the blood pressure. Hence blood pressure measurement is not always undertaken with the primary intention of assessing the blood pressure level. The difficulty in recent years though is that if a doctor takes a blood pressure as a symbolic routine he may feel constrained, by the uncritical acceptance and unwarranted status of theoretical medical knowledge, to record a level in the range of 90-110 diastolic as raised, and so diagnose hypertension and institute long term treatment. So far from being a source of optimism and reassurance the symbolic routine may acquire serious diagnostic implications almost by accident. Opportunistic screening may also produce unintended and unfortunate results, because if all adult patients have their blood pressure taken as an automatic part of every consultation, there can be no place for the selection of certain patients for blood pressure measurement. The possibility of symbolic routines having any personal meaning is negated once the procedure involved becomes the subject of universal screening, because they have become replaced by a solely technical task.

By the end of the 1980s a number of largescale trials involving several countries had been completed and the British Hypertension Working Party concluded from a review of them that:

> On the basis of existing evidence we suggest that drug treatment is indicated in men and women under 80 where diastolic blood pressure averages 100mm Hg over three to four months.(14)

Two relevant points can be noted from this. First that the level of blood pressure finally recommended for treatment was not as low as some authorities had predicted and on the basis of which they had established trials. Second even after all the evidence had been considered no attention whatever was paid to the personal and symbolic qualities referred to here. Within the medical research community they are either not considered at all, or are not seen as having any relevance to the research process. Decisions about the diagnosis and treatment of high blood pressure are therefore dealt with as if they are entirely a matter to be decided by a technical research procedure. There is no sense in which symbolic and personal qualities can impinge on this, either in the conceptualisation of the condition itself, or in influencing the research method. Their only possible role is as something to be considered after the technical rationale has been finalised.

There are further difficulties which arise with research involving screening, especially where what is being treated is one amongst a number of risk factors which may or may not be of importance in an individual case, where the subject has never experienced any symptoms, and where prevention is a long-term strategy. To begin with there is an assumption that the pathological process will remain stable, so that the subjects of the research will experience an identical disease process to the reference subjects to which the research is applied. When the research concerns short-term treatment, the experimental and reference subjects are likely to be similar in most relevant respects, so the assumption will hold. However when the research may take five or ten years to complete, and then be applied to a population where the preventive strategy is expected to unfold over twenty or more years, there may be considerable biological divergence between the experimental and reference subjects, such that the calculation about risks may not hold good.

In addition to this attempting to identify, quantify and aggregate costs and benefits, as is required if a formula is to be used in determining whether intervention is deemed 'worthwhile', is particularly problematic. It is well known that doctors have great difficulty in persuading people who feel perfectly well that they are at risk of serious disease at some future time that may be many years hence. So what doctors regard as a major and worthwhile benefit of prevention needs itself to be evaluated, taking into account that it may be of relatively little concern or relevance to the person involved. On the other hand if that person does take it seriously, he is likely to view himself differently in having accepted that he has the medical disorder, hypertension; and though he does not feel unwell, this may have a significant social and psychological effect on his life. To such a person this may represent an important cost that has been incurred by diagnosis and treatment, but the doctor will be likely to play it down, stressing that the point of prevention is the maintenance of a normal healthy state, and he will draw attention to the lowered blood pressure as evidence. The point here is that there are no unequivocal criteria by which such differences of perspective can be resolved, because the resort of the positivist to objective medical knowledge, to be upheld and applied by doctors, has been shown to be unacceptable. Therefore without any straightforward means by which to even identify and agree on the nature of all the costs and benefits in a particular case, the task of quantifying and aggregating them becomes even more problematic. Then because these factors also change with time the picture is further compounded.

What emerges from this is that in such long-term trials of prevention involving the alteration of risk factors, the built-in biomedical assumptions are not well-founded, so that the results from these studies are much less accurate than is generally claimed. Further than this, the personal and social differences associated with the identification and summation of costs and benefits makes the whole basis of the research still more tenuous. It is not just that it adds to the biomedical imprecision, which would be serious enough, but that the two aspects of this double uncertainty, the biomedical and the personal/social interact with each other. The personal worry likely to be associated with being labelled a hypertensive, and the current social understanding of what it is to have such a medical condition, will themselves lead to biomedical changes which may be relevant to the development of cardiovascular disease; but it is not possible to predict how all these changes will progress, or be seen by the different parties involved.

None of this should be taken as suggesting that the clinical and symbolic aspects of medicine are mutually exclusive, or that the relationship between them should never change. What is at issue is the unquestioning pursuit of technological rationalism, which has led to the suppression and distortion of the symbolic element. Hence the need for a reappraisal which gives due weight to the two sides and how they should relate to each other.

Some years ago Dollery, a prominent member of the medical establishment, reviewed the state of western medicine, and observed that there was a paradox in that we seem to have come to the end of an age of optimism, despite what he saw as the increasingly successful application of technology.(15) Not surprisingly he concluded that the only substantial criticism that needed serious attention was that of Cochrane which requires stricter dedication to research assessment especially through the use of the RCT. But this fails to address the paradox because it contains two conflicting messages. On the one hand progress in medicine is regarded as reliant on a technical process which is morally neutral, and not something about which either optimism or pessimism is appropriate. On the other hand the idea of medical progress as something which addresses human needs, contains within it the notion of optimism.

The pervasive feeling of disillusionment about the direction of western medicine and technology in general, is therefore not something which can be dismissed simply by reference to the neutrality of technology. The medical scientist cannot ally himself with the almost universal yearning for progress in improving health care and at the same time deny that his methods are implicated when that longing by the public is not fulfilled in a way that he feels to be appropriate. Part of the problem is that the oversimplistic identification of medical technology with progress has so long been widely shared by the public and the medical profession, that the latter feel understandably betrayed when this vision is no longer shared. This is not to suggest that many of the benefits of medical technology should be denied or dismissed; what is required though is a recognition that the status that has become conferred on technology was always flawed, and that recent difficulties merely demonstrate this more clearly than before. Seen in this way the achievements of medical technology and research as well as the aura which surrounds them, have been the victims of their own success, because whilst the public remained uncritically enthusiastic the professional leaders were only too willing to swallow their own propaganda. Now that the public is more sceptical and ambivalent about technology, it is time the professional elite stopped trying to convince itself that nothing fundamental needs to be changed.

What medical progress signifies needs to be rethought. But without any alternative goal or personal and social sense of meaning in medicine, a false optimism continues to attach very readily to individual technical developments. Hence it is only through replacing the current worn out ideology, that technology and research will appear in a different light. One way of identifying and challenging this position is to acknowledge the importance of reassessing the role of optimism and trust in medicine and health care, by dislocating their almost exclusive association with technology and research.

What role is then left for medical technology and research in future? First of all the different view of their status presented here does not allow any final and definitive statement about this, only some positive indications as to the right direction. An awareness of the inevitability of differences of interpretation about

126

the benefits of technology should lead to a much greater humility and caution in advancing and proceeding with new technical procedures and treatments. It should also lead to a much more thoroughgoing reappraisal of technology already in use, and a greater willingness to stop or revise it. This does not invalidate the generally accepted techniques of research, but places a different emphasis on how and when they should be used, and what conclusions can be drawn from them. The status accorded to the RCT in particular will be changed and diminished.

This generally more cautious attitude to technology would then allow for and be paralleled by the greater recognition of and importance placed on the personal and symbolic elements of medicine. Thus the meaning of medical progress would become redefined in terms of both sustaining medical technology in future and of carrying forward medicine and health care as a human enterprise, which would include a genuine and realistic prospect for optimism for all the parties concerned.

10 A different approach to the goals of health care and the implications for resource allocation

Of all the problems currently facing medicine and health care in western societies, the most serious and intractable is usually thought to be that of resource allocation - how to distribute finite resources in the face of ever-increasing demands for health care. The paradox is that spending on health care in western countries has been rising both in real terms and as a proportion of their GNP for many years, and yet far from going away the problem is seen to be getting worse. So resource allocation difficulties have become viewed as one of the penalties of the success of modern medicine, and in recent years the issue has spawned a large literature, offering a variety of approaches as to how it should be tackled in practical, moral and political terms. In this chapter it will be shown that almost all this effort has been based on certain assumptions about the nature and goals of health care, which have already been challenged but have not yet been related to the question of resource allocation. It will then be suggested that there is a tradition in British medicine, which taken together with the critique of western medicine that has been developed here, can be built on so as to redirect attention away from the usual preoccupations of those concerned with resource allocation.

The establishment of the NHS in Britain in 1948 was a unique achievement not followed by any other country at that time, which beside the political will required a confident leap of imagination, not least as to how such a system could hope to find the resources to fulfil the demand. Until then state intervention in relation to medicine and health care had been directed to two main goals; the pursuit of the public good and the improvement of individual health. By the 1930s a number of services had developed to fulfil these functions but in a piecemeal fashion. These included those provided by the local authorities who had taken over the Poor Law hospitals, administered the many public health acts, and provided maternal and child health services, as well as the mental and infectious diseases hospitals. In addition there was the National Insurance scheme which was introduced in 1912 and covered general practitioner services. What the NHS envisaged, which was wholly new, was that the twin goals of public and individual good in medicine and health care could

129

be maximised in such a way as to complement one another within a single affordable system. In doing so it incorporated what had traditionally been regarded as opposing ideas, those of public efficiency and rationality on the one hand and of equity and comprehensiveness on the other. It had previously been considered that to provide free services for all those in need of health care, would open the floodgates to such levels of demand that no publicly funded system could contemplate such a step. The principles of the NHS were then thought to resolve two problems simultaneously, that of a potential clash between public and individual health care goals, and that of resource allocation by the provision of state funds to fulfil all health care needs. Therefore the intention was to eliminate the need to consider resource allocation questions, and it was expected that this would hold good for all time.

Now it is the assumptions embedded within this understanding of the NHS which have formed the basis from which the debate about health care policy has proceeded ever since. And it will be contended that the current concerns about resource allocation are usually framed, either explicitly or implicitly, by these original assumptions from which a simple economic formula can be derived which then determines the questions which are posed. It relates supply and demand to an ideal model in the following way:

The total resources required when managed with maximum efficiency = The cost of the best care in relation to total health care needs

There were a number of reasons why the original architects of the NHS considered that the government could afford to live with this formulation. First because they thought that centralised state provision would be more efficient and better managed than a set of disparate services which could not be satisfactorily co-ordinated. Second that total health care needs and the cost of best care were viewed as determinate entities which were specifiable at any given time. Third that total health care needs would diminish with progress in medical technology and optimal care, although it was also foreseen that this would be offset by increases in the cost of improvement in care. Thus in the Beveridge Report published in 1942, it was stated in estimating the cost of the planned health service that:

No change is made in this figure as from 1945-1965, it being assumed that there will actually be some development of the service, and as a consequence of the development a reduction in the number of cases requiring it.(1)

Despite the fact that from the very beginning doubts were expressed about the increasing costs of the NHS and the ability of the government to meet them,(2) the original perception that the system was workable was widely shared during the first twenty years of the service, and so the question of resource allocation was not raised as an important and serious economic and political issue during that time. It was generally accepted that the broad principles of the NHS were compatible with a reasonable and affordable level of costs based on the economic formulation given above. So the NHS was seen to be economically viable and indefinitely sustainable given the political will. By the 1970s, though, escalating medical technology, coupled with increasing demands and national economic difficulties, led to a changed climate in which resource allocation questions came to the fore and have been central to policy debates ever since. This shift was marked by the emergence of the subdiscipline of health economics whose principle concern derived from the new interest in the allocation of scarce resources.

The purpose now is to analyse how this change in perception has been conceptualised in relation to the original economic formulation. Since 1970 there have been four major reorganisations of the NHS (in 1974, 1982, 1984 and 1991) which reflect this change. They have all been directed towards improving management efficiency (although I have argued elsewhere that the 1991 reorganisation involving the creation of an internal market can be interpreted differently(3)), and each with limited success, so that further reorganisation, and yet more attempts to improve efficiency have been seen as the main solution. One way of viewing this succession of organisational upheavals is to see them as ostensibly addressing the question of resource allocation, but actually not confronting it in practice, partly by claiming that management efficiency will avoid the need to do so, and partly through a wish to deny that it need be faced at all. Constantly focusing on the supply side of the economic formula by claiming that management efficiency is the key to controlling costs may function so as to distract attention away from a more fundamental reassessment of the demand components of the formula. Hence what has been left unquestioned is the status of health care needs and the meaning of best care. It has been assumed that at any given time they are fixed and hence can only be dealt with by meeting them in full or in terms of rationing. The reluctance of the public, health care professionals and politicians to conduct an open debate about this whole area is then an inhibition to the consideration of alternative approaches. What follows is therefore a detailed exploration of the unexamined assumptions concerning health care needs and best care. This will involve a reassessment of ideas about demand and supply in relation to health care, such that resource allocation questions are no longer seen to be of primary concern.

Turning to health care needs first, western medicine has come to interpret them within the context of a positivist and reductionist conception of medical knowledge defined in technical terms. Now if we consider that a comprehensive understanding of medicine and health care encompasses a number of broad goals, this conception of medical knowledge can only be readily related to one of them - the technical management of diseases, disability and injury. Other goals, notably the personal care and support of the sick and the improvement of the general health of the population, tend to be either excluded or dealt with in such a way as to distort them. So it is only through this restrictive interpretation that it is possible to view health care needs as factual and potentially able to be completely determined. Hence for a given population it is seen to be theoretically possible to list and aggregate the total of health care needs. They are then regarded as naturally occurring and empirically describable, and so discoverable by doctors or other appropriate health care professionals, by reference to a body of publicly available medical knowledge.

What this theoretical notion hides though, is that in practice health care needs are not so readily or exhaustively delineated and are open to dispute. So there are always varying opinions as to whether certain needs should fall within the realm of health care e.g. those arising from alcoholism and infertility; and as to whether other issues which have been conceived in terms of health care needs can change culturally and historically e.g. homosexuality and mental handicap. According to the traditional view such differences of opinion and changes can only be interpreted as mistakes which arise from a lack of knowledge and therefore are correctable. However, as previously described, a more rounded and adequate understanding of medicine and health care and thus of health care needs is not amenable to such a ready and precise agreed definition. Even when there is agreement at this theoretical level, there can still be disputes about whether particular individuals qualify as having particular health care needs, and once again conventional wisdom is that they are resolvable by reference to technical expertise. So the proposal made by Evans 'to influence and in some sense limit the actual or perceived health needs of the population'(4) in attempting to deal with the demand for health care makes no sense on the traditional interpretation of need. On this view demand and need for health care can always be brought into line because the doctor is regarded as the legitimate and final arbiter. However it is precisely increasing demand for health care, over and above increasing health care need (due to demographic change and burgeoning technology), which is often cited as a significant reason for the rise in health care costs in recent years, and hence the necessity for resource allocation. So once again there would seem to be a tension between theory and practice.

Returning then to a consideration of the early years of the NHS the opposite claim is usually made about that period, namely that disputes about discrepancies between demands and needs rarely occurred, and this helped doctors to keep costs low. However it is also generally accepted that this was because doctors acted paternalistically in not discussing the situation with patients, thereby preventing them from making demands and so limiting the definition of health care needs. Whilst this may have been partly true, it obscures other important facets of the situation. At that time patients and the public generally, rarely sought to challenge doctors, and so tacitly accepted the definition of health care needs provided. It was not so much that patients' views were always the same as their doctors, as that there was a shared culture in which challenges to the doctor's authority were not usually expected by either doctors or patients. In addition there is no reason to assume that the view taken by doctors of health care needs at that time had any privileged status in a positivist sense.

Therefore it could be argued that the early years of the NHS were characterised by a non-inflationary culture in which health care needs were determined by a social process which, by and large, was a continuation of a previous pattern. Before 1948 the principal services for the provision of personal health care for the majority of the population were those administered by the local authorities (some of which had derived from the Poor Law), the voluntary charitable hospitals and the National Insurance scheme in relation to general practice. All these various services had one thing in common, that health care needs were defined by doctors who were encouraged to apply a restrictive rather than a liberal interpretation of what that meant in practice. The gradual change in definition of health care needs in recent years is not then from an accepted and unchallenged positivist definition, to a positivist definition under pressure from consumer demand. Instead it is properly seen as a transition from one socially derived conception of health care needs to a different one, in which both lay and professional perspectives are necessarily involved in each period. Further, the extent of this transition shows considerable variation between countries, with Britain having changed less than many other western countries. As Payer observed as recently as 1990 'The most striking characteristic of British medicine is its economy. The British do less of nearly everything'.(5)

Therefore the conclusion to be drawn from this consideration of health care needs is that they are traditionally conceived in theoretical terms as capable of being exactly and objectively determined, and so specifiable at any given time, but that this is a false and seriously distorting notion. They are in fact defined in social and political terms, within the constraints of certain moral limits. It is not that health care needs are culturally relative concepts, with virtually unlimited variations between different societies, but that there will inevitably be certain inter-societal variations whose acceptability can only be determined by moral reflection and judgement. Seen in this way it becomes apparent that health care needs are not fixed points around which moral arguments can be constructed, but are themselves matters of moral debate. The nature of traditional concerns about resource allocation has therefore to be altered, making them only a secondary consideration, and the importance of this different understanding is crucial in refocusing the whole debate.

The other main issue concerns the interpretation of best care in medicine, and it will be suggested once again that the traditional conception is flawed in a manner that parallels that described in relation to health care needs. In recent times the uncritical acceptance of the apparently irresistible logic of western medicine has been such that for both the public and the medical profession, a general rule has come to be widely accepted that more diagnosis and intervention is usually better, and less is usually worse. The United States has probably taken this the furthest, with Britain some way behind, although it is only a matter of degree. In fact this attitude is so prevalent and taken for granted, that for many it is an article of faith which affects medical practice across the board. Scheff, an American sociologist, described this process some years ago in relation to diagnosis, and formulated it as a decision rule that doctors generally follow '... judging a sick person well is more to be avoided than judging a well person sick'.(6) So on the whole doctors prefer to err towards overdiagnosing than underdiagnosing disease, and are more concerned not to miss a disease than to wrongly diagnose disease.

A difference in practice which reflects a different emphasis can be noted here between the U.S. and Britain. In the U.S. it is usual for patients to have direct access to medical specialists, and they may see several about a single complaint, all of whom will initiate their own investigations. So, following Scheff's rule, they are most likely, when taken collectively, to reach a diagnosis or more than one diagnosis. In Britain on the other hand, patients seen within the NHS can only be referred to specialists by their general practitioner, who monitors their overall care and will rarely refer them to more than one specialist for a particular episode of illness. Unlike the U.S. it is also rare in Britain for patients to have special investigations carried out before they have been assessed by the doctor. Equally the ordering of batteries of tests, rather than carrying them out sequentially, is more common in the U.S. than Britain, although this practice is gaining ground everywhere as automation becomes increasingly available. It would seem then that one aspect of Scheff's decision rule could be formulated as follows - 'If in doubt carry out special investigations', because to omit a test is regarded as a more serious error than not to do so, although the system of general practice in Britain remains a strong counter to this overall trend.

In general terms this same thinking can also be applied to treatment. Much has been made in recent years about the importance of obtaining the patient's informed consent to all treatment decisions, and patients undoubtedly have more possibility of influencing their treatment than they did a generation ago. But what is less often considered is the context in which such decisions are made. What is presented to patients is usually the considered opinion of the doctor as to what is best, and this is characteristically towards intervention, and often aggressive intervention, rather than a more cautious approach. The model the doctor believes he is using is one which embodies the idea of objective best treatment and care, which it would be wrong for him not to offer the patient as his preferred option. But such a view far from being neutral, is typically framed by a bias in favour of intervention, and the degree and direction of this bias varies considerably even between western countries. The relevant point is that both doctors and patients in a particular society share a common understanding that there is a clear definition of what constitutes best treatment and care, and that a positive stance towards the use of technical intervention is usually regarded as the right approach. So it is not surprising that the occasions on which patients withhold their consent to proposed treatments, or have any real wish to consider doing so, are fairly limited.

A hypothetical example will now be constructed, to illustrate in more specific terms how important the medical decision-making process is in determining the degree of technical content and intervention which results. The case to be considered concerns a young woman who lost two stones in weight over a six month period, with dull abdominal pain during the later three months. Her mother had died of stomach cancer in middle age. She had been separated from her husband for a year, had no children and worked as a secretary.

There are a number of critical points in the decision-making process related to this case, of which three of the most important will be considered here, as they might arise in the British context:

(1) Self-referral to the general practitioner:
  (a) as soon as weight loss begins;
  (b) when abdominal pain begins, three months later;
  (c) when weight loss is substantial and abdominal pain continues, six months later.
(2) Decisions taken by the general practitioner after the initial consultation:
  (a) reassurance and follow-up;
  (b) arrangements for special investigations;
  (c) referral to a physician;
  (d) referral to a surgeon;
  (e) referral for psychological assessment.
(3) Decisions taken by the specialist after the initial consultation:
  (a) whether to order special investigations and how many; and whether to order them as a block or sequentially;
  (b) whether to start treatment immediately, and if so what kind, e.g. medical, surgical or psychological.

From this relatively simple example it can be seen that a range of different decision-making choices are available at each of these three levels, and that the selection of different options will have very different implications for the use that is made of technology, particularly as the decisions made are cumulative. The possibility for overall variation is therefore very great, and consistent biases towards certain patterns of decision-making will have major implications for the use of technology and the costs of any health care system. On the whole though the general tendency within western medicine is to favour technical processes and intervention.

An important aspect of this situation is that what is viewed as medical error has become distorted, so that all error in medicine has come to be regarded as technical error:

> It is assumed apparently that patients get sick from diseases from which they can be cured. If they are not cured, or if they are given treatments, medical or surgical, which are unnecessary or do them harm, then error has been committed. Such error, the assumption seems to be, is technical in nature and thus always knowable.(7)

What there is no room for is a recognition that western medicine does not and cannot encompass a complete technical package capable of defining for each case what best treatment and care consists of. So there is no place for what might be called symbolic error, rather than technical error. Strictly, symbolic error is not error at all but more accurately poor judgement. This can never be eliminated altogether in any system which is beset by inherent uncertainties, but it can be in part through the exercise of better judgement.

Given this situation of incomplete information and changing circumstances the line between technical and symbolic error is not entirely clear, and the best judgements may sometimes turn out to have bad outcomes, whilst favourable outcomes may sometimes stem from poor judgements. Hence judgement cannot be tied to 'successful' and predicted outcomes, and other means must be found to assess what constitutes good practice. What is required is a balance between a degree of professional autonomy in the specification of standards of practice, and an external review by legal regulation as well as by community involvement e.g. through ethical committees and consumer groups.

In Britain institutional mechanisms such as these are already in place, but they are restricted in their operation by the collective understanding of what is involved. The problem is that the ideology of western medicine tends to allow for only one interpretation as Cassell explains:

> However, I believe the greatest source of error lies in the inherent belief and value structure of medicine, equally shared, as must be the case, by both physicians and patients. Where the belief exists that fate in its expression as illness can be denied or overcome, and where the cure is the expectation, there exists a force to act. Medicine is based on a belief in the efficacy of intervention.(8)

Now if western medicine is indeed based on a belief in the efficacy of technical intervention, then a bias towards technical action as producing best treatment and care becomes imperative, and when it fails in technical terms will tend to be seen as technical error. Only a change in understanding of the place of technology in medicine can alter this and make possible a different perspective in which best treatment and care can be evaluated in other ways. Such a change would then open the door to the possibility of judging technical processes and interventions at all stages with a more sceptical eye. The ideal of best care would lose its sense of precision, by dispensing with the ideology that constantly strains towards the notion that more technology is necessarily better.

Two traditional and central ideas, of health care needs and best care, have now been challenged and alternative perspectives have been presented in each case. What also needs to be recognised is that these criticisms are inter-related because the underlying concern applies to both of them. This is that the definition of health care needs and best care is not solely a technical matter which is therefore readily specifiable, but is also social and moral and so necessarily a matter of judgement, no matter what arrangements are made in the exercise of that judgement. In addition although health care needs and best care have been analysed as if they were separate matters, in practice what are considered health care needs tend to be influenced by the technical care available, and what is regarded as best care is itself influenced by ideas of what constitute health care needs. So for example, the recent growth in new technologies relevant to assisted conception has itself framed much of the debate as to whether assisted conception should be regarded as a health care need, and also of what best care might mean in this context.

Concepts of health care needs and of best care are therefore interactive, and when considered jointly give rise to a rather diffuse and malleable notion of what the total of best medical care for any population consists of. Therefore it should not come as a surprise that the treatment and care actually provided by different societies, even with the same resources available, differs quite markedly, because there is no single and exact template against which to evaluate what any system provides. This realisation may appear at first to lead to insurmountable problems in developing health policy because of the indeterminacy of the available building blocks. But the less concrete and more open ideas being suggested can be viewed instead as presenting a different and new opportunity. This is because they raise the possibility of breaking away from the fundamental belief in forever advancing medical technology as an imperative. Health policy then becomes subject to moral judgements which are not pre-empted and so driven by an overriding reliance on the supremacy of technology. This being so the spectre of the inevitability of inflationary health care costs running out of control because of technology, no longer has to follow. There is the prospect of formulating what are judged to be good and appropriate health care policies which derive from a non-inflationary medical culture. The question though is can we and should we be doing anything to facilitate this culture?

Once the idealisation of the role of technology in medicine has been set aside it is clear that different health policies could be developed, and equally making choices about the direction to be taken would be unavoidable. Whereas previously the way ahead seemed mapped out in advance, a new direction has now been opened up which requires that judgements and choices be made. On the old assumptions ever-increasing inflationary pressures must at some point be met by demands that limits are set, and the question of how to allocate resources then becomes the most fundamental issue in all decisions relating to health policy. The alternative scenario removes the primacy focus away from resource allocation to question the appropriateness of any postulated goal of health policy. This does not mean that a shortage of resources and hence allocation will never have to be considered, but these issues no longer dominate the agenda, because they only arise at a secondary stage. The new perspective allows for positive evaluation to be made about health policy, rather than the negative and reactive process entailed by the denial of services arising through policies of resource allocation.

One indication of how to conceptualise this change has been suggested by ten Have, and involves a switch from a policy that sets limits to health care to one about making choices.(9) The latter he sees as encouraging and reasserting what he regards as the fundamental principles of equal access and solidarity in health care. Following this line of reasoning it could be argued that the early years of the NHS in Britain were characterised by the widespread acceptance of these principles, and that it was this which gave rise to a shared culture in which inflationary pressures were largely resisted. There should be no sense of denying the misconceptions and problems which existed in this period, but it does draw attention to the need for the reassertion of moral values in the definition of health policy, rather than merely as a response to demographic and technical developments.

This type of analysis shifts attention away from the notion of best care to be strained after and only relinquished with reluctance, to that of right or appropriate care in any particular set of social or political circumstances. There is then the risk of being charged with evading problems of the adequacy of resources, but this is not the intention and is quite different from being drawn inevitably into a situation of spiralling costs. Equally it does not sanction poor levels of care, nor suggest that there has ever been a golden era when services were wholly appropriate and admirable, but it does allow that choosing to do less than is technically possible may not only be a reasonable approach but the right one. The difficult questions then arise as to how to make such judgements and on what basis.

Serious debates about these issues have already begun in relation to the use of technology at the end of life, and where life is deemed futile,(10) but they have not yet been articulated in a comprehensive manner so as to apply to medicine as a whole. The intention behind the arguments presented here has been to provide the background on which a more complete analysis could be built, and in so doing to draw attention away from the current preoccupation with resource allocation, towards an appreciation of both the need and the possibility of re-evaluating the goals of health care once they are freed from unreflective obeisance to the idol of technological progress. What is required as a precondition of bringing this about, is not in the first instance a change in institutional arrangements, but a different awareness on all sides (amongst health care professionals, the public and the government) of the failure of past assumptions and a preparedness to rethink them. Some proposals as to what this would entail will be made in the concluding chapter.

11 Conclusion

The purpose of this concluding chapter is two-fold. First to return to and develop some of the themes concerning the meaning of mystery in relation to medicine which were introduced and discussed in the first chapter. Second to draw together some of the theoretical and practical implications that have been explored in the body of the thesis, in order to show how when taken jointly, they form the framework for a critique of western medicine as a whole. This is not to suggest that all aspects of western medicine have been considered, but that a way of doing so has been set out. As the analysis has been mainly of the operation of western medicine within the developed world, some additional observations will be made about its relevance to medicine in developing countries.

In chapter one a number of suggestions were made as to the role of mystery in western medicine, and in the course of the arguments which were developed subsequently the focus has continually returned to a conception of mystery involving an inescapable element of indeterminacy and uncertainty in all aspects of medicine. Therefore the first part of this chapter will explore in more detail what such an understanding entails.

In considering the original distinctions made in chapter one between mystery as a potentially soluble puzzle and mystery involving an inescapable element of indeterminacy and uncertainty, it is important to recognise that the former does not diminish the latter. This is because although part of what is presently obscure may prove to be knowable in future, other facets of the unknown will become apparent at the same time. It is not so much that we can identify particular areas which are essentially opaque and so forever resistant to understanding, but that new and often unpredictable circumstances concerning the unknown will always be arising. Included in this must be that what are thought of at present as certainties, may themselves become uncertain. The salient point then is that indeterminacy and uncertainty are general features of all medical knowledge and understanding, not something attaching to specific designated areas.

However this insight regarding the pervasiveness of uncertainty contrasts with the common desire to create and cling to conditions which allow for a feeling of certainty in medicine, so denying a role for mystery, and this partly derives from the prevalent misunderstanding that mystery implies irrationality and obscurity. The fear is then of scepticism as to man's ability to improve health and control disease. However this does not follow, because what is meant by mystery is more subtle and adds further realms to the understanding of mystery than have been considered so far. Laurens van der Post expressed one aspect of this in his biography of Jung:

> Mystery includes the known as well as the unknown; the ordinary as well as the extraordinary. Once the feeling of mystery abandons our travel-stained senses in contemplation of the same well-worn scene, we have ceased, in some vital sense, to know what we are observing.(1)

So far from obscuring understanding, mystery is an essential part of it. Therefore recognising the role of mystery is not in opposition to clarity of understanding. Improving knowledge and understanding must always involve dealing with those elements of uncertainty which can be resolved, but the notion of mystery goes beyond this to touch on a different dimension which is beyond any final resolution.

Another insight was suggested by Wisdom in his book *Paradox and Discovery* when he proposed that in seeking knowledge the way of dealing with uncertainty and bewilderment is inevitably problematic:

> The trouble is that the concepts, without which we do not connect one thing with another, are apt to become a network which confines our minds. We need to be at once like someone who has seen much and forgotten nothing, and also like one who is seeing everything for the first time.(2)

So improved comprehension and understanding require both great experience and an innocence of approach, and this produces a tension that can never be completely resolved. However it is one of the hallmarks of wise physicians that they attempt to embody a combination of these two characteristics.

It is not simply a question of knowing that something is the case, but also of how and why. For example we may know with a degree of certainty that someone has a terminal condition, but little of why the condition has affected them, and even less of how they come to understand and cope with their own death. The issue of knowledge for whom and from what perspective relates to this and is also of relevance. The viewpoint of patients and professionals will necessarily differ, and the recognition of that difference is an acknowledgement of the need for empathetic understanding; but also of the impossibility of closing the gap between them altogether, which it itself an expression of the mystery of the relationship.

Medical systems of knowledge are therefore torn between the desire for 'closure' which will allow for diagnosis of disease, clinical research and technical control, and the 'openness' of experiential reality arising from an engagement with the patients' illnesses and suffering. However attempts to integrate and so fully comprehend these two aspects can only be partially successful. Yet at the same time in making the attempt to hold them together we engage with reality, and thereby alter it.

What emerges from these varied perspectives is a richer and multifaceted view of medical knowledge and mystery, in which the notion of necessary indeterminacy remains central, but is expanded and fleshed out in subtle and complex ways. However there is a serious difficulty in being able to demonstrate the richness of this understanding because very few authors writing about western medicine ever refer to the notion of mystery, and so the issues are difficult to discern except tangentially. Horobin's article entitled 'Professional Mystery: The Maintenance of Charisma in General Practice' is a rare exception, and the use of the word mystery in a medical article is so unusual that it indicates how alien a notion it is in relation to scientific medicine. Why though should Horobin be concerned with mystery? He suggests that it is because:

> ... mystery surrounds especially those crafts which seem to shape our world and deal with matters which seem beyond our control and comprehension. Medicine and Science with a capital 'S' are perhaps the most obvious examples of such esoteric worlds.(3)

This introduces the further paradox that on the one hand mystery is universal in the affairs of men, but on the other hand has a particular and special relationship with certain areas such as medicine and science. However, with respect to medicine, it is less of a paradox than it seems at first, because there is no suggestion that the relationship between mystery and medicine is unique, it is just that issues of medicine and health care are of such central importance in shaping our lives and also so often seem beyond our control and understanding. One aspect of this is that no entirely satisfactory definition of health is possible, because the different strands involved are themselves open to different interpretations and cannot be completely harmonised. An example is the tension between definitions of health which are holistic and concentrate on positive qualities and those which are reductionist and restrictive concentrating on the elimination of negative qualities. Beyond this these general conceptualisations are themselves expressed in a great variety of ways within different medical traditions. So the range of meanings that are encompassed by such an important and complex notion as health are inexhaustible and under constant revision and reinterpretation. Hence medicine poses questions relevant to the notion of mystery in a more heightened manner than is usual elsewhere. Equally an awareness of mystery in medicine brings with it an acceptance that no description or definition of health could ever be entirely finalised, even in principle.

One important conclusion which follows from this understanding of medical knowledge, is that it is not simply a subset of scientific knowledge in general, as would be the case if it were interpreted in terms of a positivist conception of science. Hence Wartofsky raises the following question:

Is medical knowledge to fashion itself in the image of an ideal norm of general rationality (presumably that of "science" proper or of "the scientific method"), or is medicine instead one of the constitutive cognitive practices which contributes to the very formulation of this norm itself? Put in this way, the question is no longer simply "How can medicine become scientific?" but also and perhaps more significantly, "What does an examination of the nature of medical knowledge contribute to a deeper and more adequate conception of scientific knowledge and of human knowledge more generally?"(4)

What may be drawn from this is that medical knowledge cannot be separated and insulated from other sources of knowledge, but rather is in perpetual interaction with them. Hence medical knowledge is not only a subject for investigation, but also has a role in creating and comprehending the whole realm of scientific and human knowledge.

Toulmin has also addressed this issue more recently, and in reaching a similar conclusion has developed it in a different direction to show that current distinctions between organic and psychosomatic disease, and between somatic medicine and psychotherapy do not hold good:

Thus, the psychological component in clinical medicine does not represent the external intrusion of issues irrelevant to the study of pathology: rather, the discovery of organic disorder puts a physiological slant on a clinical interaction that initially takes place on a psychological plane.(5)

Hence there is a lack of clear distinction between what have been regarded traditionally as different branches of medical knowledge, as well as there being no very precise boundaries between medical and other forms of knowledge. So for both these reasons medical knowledge cannot be characterised in any exact and definitive manner. These insights have then been used in this book to show the shortcomings of the current understanding of the relationship between orthodox and alternative medicine, and of the conceptualisation of medical knowledge within such polarised categories. Following this same line of argument the methodology of medical research has also been shown to require significant modification if it is to reflect this new appraisal of the proper form and status of medical knowledge. Thus the entire theoretical basis of medicine and health care will come to be viewed in a different light as these various aspects of medical knowledge are revealed and acknowledged.

Turning now from theory to practice, the notion of mystery as it relates to individual clinical practice was explored in chapter six, and its recognition requires the humility of comprehending that 'both physician and patient are in the presence of a deep human mystery greater than both of them'.(6) The present purpose is to trace some of the implications of this in relation to the development of public policy.

The issue to be addressed is most readily understood by starting from failures which arise at the individual decision-making level:

> The doctor derives his right to ethical decision-making from the society and from the individual patient. But he and his patient protect themselves from the awesome implications of that responsibility by hiding behind the belief that doctors only make technical decisions.(7)

The doctor-patient relationship is determined by a social framework, so that the responsibilities of doctors and patients are set within a social context. However the emphasis that is placed on the individual nature of each patient contact coupled with the stress put on its being primarily technical, serve to obscure and deny this social dimension. Thus both doctor and patient are unwittingly conspiring to conceal the truth of what is happening during the consultation, and so distorting the nature of the relationship of power and responsibility that is involved. The basis of the doctor-patient encounter is therefore partly false. As Ladd observes, within any democratic system:

> ... responsibility and power are public concepts; that is, power, if anything, is or ought to be an object of public scrutiny. The first aspect of the ethics of power is accountability, that is, the person who has the power ought to be prepared to explain, justify and defend his actions and non-actions. The exercise of power without accountability is ethically unacceptable. It is irresponsible.(8)

So the failure to recognise the true nature of the individual encounter leads to a collective irresponsibility which is not readily countered because it is part and parcel of a whole system of medicine. It is not that doctors or patients set out deliberately to obscure the truth, but that the jointly held assumptions with which they operate in order to regulate exchange and expectation have been excluded from the realm where public questions of power and responsibility are seen to be relevant. In a more general analysis of what makes the modern mind Gellner proposes that 'Greater and greater expanses of truth acquire an autonomy from the social, moral and political obligations and decencies of the society'(9); and medicine and health

145

care offer prime examples of an area of life which has partially escaped from public scrutiny and so from a publicly evaluated account of their truth and meaning. Once this situation has become entrenched, all those who are involved including the professionals, the public, the managers and the government, can only apply fragmented responses to problems as they arise. This is because they all remain in thrall to a common understanding of medicine and health care, to which they are jointly committed, but which their flawed perception leaves them in no position to challenge. This determines that each of the groups concerned conceives of its responsibility in a narrow and limited way, which is difficult to transcend on either a group or a collective basis.

Only by finding the means to break into this closed circle of awareness will it be possible to see a new way forward; and an important conclusion of this thesis is the proposal that recognising the role of mystery in medicine is crucial in this respect. One aspect of this is to question the modern idea of progress. This was discussed in chapter one and is well expressed by Midgley, in relation to society generally:

> For the last three centuries, able people have been celebrating the astonishing achievements of the human intellect and the human will ... . The dominant world picture in our culture has been one of steady linear progress brought about by that will and intellect, an improvement booked to continue indefinitely. (10)

Callahan then goes further in suggesting that western medicine has clung on to this global view for longer than elsewhere:

> Medicine is perhaps the last and purist bastion of Enlightenment dreams, tying together reason, science and the dream of unlimited human possibilities. There is nothing, it is held, that in principle cannot be done and, given suitable caution, little than ought not to be done. (11)

By acknowledging the inevitability of indeterminacy and uncertainty the imperative of such progress can be challenged, and the scene is then set for a change of emphasis to a new imperative of responsibility. This would require that moral concerns took precedence, rather than coming in by way of response to technological developments which are already in place or taking shape. The importance of attempting such a moral and conceptual shift lies in its potential to overturn the old ways of thinking, by unveiling the abnegation of social responsibility which has produced a pattern of collective irresponsibility.

However accepting the role of mystery is only the starting point, new forms of medical knowledge and practice and the institutions within which they might operate in different societies must follow. What has been attempted in this book is no more than to clear a space within which there is the possibility that such new structures with their attendant choices and judgements can emerge. The purpose has been to change the terms of the debate in such a way that all those concerned with medicine and health care will themselves be enabled to envisage new goals from which they may go on to adapt the old patterns of health care and develop new ones. The first requirement in bringing about this change has been to show that the underlying rationale of western medicine is at fault, and the second has been to demonstrate the unacceptable consequences that arise from the pursuit of illusory and unrealistic goals, which are becoming increasingly apparent throughout all countries that have adopted western systems of health care. So the direction that change will need to take has been made clear, but it would be inappropriate to formulate more detailed suggestions about such changes, or as to what specific powers and responsibilities the different groups involved might adopt. This is a task for those who are directly involved.

Something will be said though about the implications for developing countries; first because they have not featured so far but are strongly implicated in much of what has been proposed; and second because the notion of mystery in medicine applies to all medical systems, and so its exploration could have an integrative role linking together the analysis as of relevance to both developed and developing countries.

None of the developing countries has been significantly involved in the historical development of western medicine as a system, and with few exceptions this remains true today. Nevertheless developing countries have come to rely increasingly on western medicine, originally as a result of western colonialism, but more recently as part of the free market ideology associated with western medical practice and technology. In almost all developing countries this has resulted in two strands of health care, that based on traditional indigenous medical systems and that on western medicine. In some countries they exist and flourish side by side, but in others western medicine has tended to squeeze out and marginalise traditional practices, because its technical achievements have given it an apparently superior role and status. One aspect of the recognition of mystery in western medicine is that it is placed on a similar footing with all other systems of medicine in the sense that the conceptual underpinnings and potential insights of all systems are to be taken seriously. The cultural importance of healing, as opposed to technical efficacy, will thereby be emphasised and more readily valued.

One of the greatest failures of western medicine as practised in most developing countries, is the adoption of spectacular and expensive high technology care for a small elite, whilst the majority of people often fail to receive even those simple measures which could produce dramatic improvements in the general health of the population. The reasons for this are complex, and are not amenable to simple or ready made solutions, but a more critical approach to the role of technology in medicine in developed countries, will help in fostering a similar attitude in developing countries. This is not to deny the enormous need for improvements in material wealth in these societies, but to accept that as they accrue they should not be devoted largely to high technology procedures, which can only be made available to a privileged minority and even then may not be sustainable in the longterm. Thus the concept of mystery in medicine may be used to highlight related problems in both developed and developing countries, especially in directing concern to the escalation of technology, and so enables a joint agenda in the search for new solutions.

When considered on a wider canvas relations between developed and developing countries represent arguably the greatest challenge to the world as a whole, and medicine is an important part of that relationship. If the general relationship is to prosper, with developing countries growing in material wealth, there may well come a time when economic growth in developed countries will have to slow or reverse. The acceptance of mystery in western medicine would allow for the accommodation of such a change, without there being seen to be disastrous and insurmountable consequences for the health care systems of the developed world. Equally this would be an important signal for developing countries as to how they should respond to western medicine, and its related pharmaceutical and technical industries, by showing greater caution and more discrimination. The importance of such changes for medicine and health care worldwide can hardly be overstated, and the ideas developed here in relation to mystery should hasten this prospect.

In summary, mystery has been shown to be an inevitable feature of medicine and health care, and the main focus in this book has concerned the indeterminacy which is a pervasive and enduring aspect of all medical knowledge and understanding. This gives rise to a profound sense of uncertainty and awe, which can never by dispelled by the resolution of particular puzzling issues through advances in science and technology. Hence all medical endeavour is fragile and insecure, but the perception of this has been gradually eroded over the last two centuries. Regaining it is therefore a necessary corrective to the illusory and ultimately destructive goals which are presently being pursued by western medicine. Once an appreciation of the essential role of mystery has been recaptured, western medicine will be revitalised by a new awareness of its history and practice, as well as by being more open to the wisdom embodied in other systems of medicine. What is required is a new frame of reference determined by a different set of values and attitudes. This revival will then enable the growing and apparently insurmountable problems of western health care systems to be viewed in a different and more positive light. It will provide a wellspring from which it will be possible collectively to develop more sustainable and morally defensible systems of medicine.

References and notes

Chapter 2

1. Hausheer, R., 'Introduction' to Berlin, I., *Against the Current. Essays in the History of Ideas* (London: The Hogarth Press), 1979, p.xviii.
2. *The Concise Oxford Dictionary* 6th Ed. (Oxford: OUP), 1976.
3. Bergman, A.B., Beckwith, J.B. and Ray, C.G. (eds), *Proceedings of the Second International Conference on Causes of Sudden Death in Infants* (Seattle and London: University of Washington Press), 1970, p.ix.
4. *Ibid.*, p.14.
5. Reiser, S.J., *Medicine and the Reign of Technology* (Cambridge: Cambridge University Press), 1978, p.175.
6. *Ibid.*, p.176.
7. Gordon, D.R., 'Clinical Science and Clinical Expertise: Changing Boundaries Between Art and Science in Medicine' in Lock, M. and Gordon, D.R. (eds), *Biomedicine Examined* (Dordrecht: Kluwer Academic Publishers), 1988.
8. Parsons, T., *The Social System* (London: Tavistock in collaboration with Routledge and Kegan Paul), 1952, p.469 (first published Glencoe, Ill.: Free Press, 1951).
9. Malinowski, B., *Magic, Science, Religion and Other Essays* (New York: Doubleday Anchor Books), 1925, p.90 (in 1954 edition).
10. Leach, E., *Culture and Communication* (Cambridge: Cambridge University Press), 1976, p.29.
11. *Ibid.*, p.29.
12. Malinowski, B., *op.cit.*, 1925, p.90 (in 1954 edition).
13. Douglas, M., *Purity and Danger - An Analysis of Pollution and Taboo* (London: Routledge and Kegan Paul), 1966.
14. Posner, T.R., *A System of Medical Control: The Case of Diabetes* (PhD Thesis: University of London), 1989, p.297.
15. *Ibid.*, p.307.

16. Harré, R., *The Philosophies of Science* (London Oxford and New York: Oxford University Press), 1972, p.180.
17. Ryan, A., *The Philosophy of the Social Sciences* (London and Basingstoke: Macmillan and Co.Ltd.), 1970, p.204.
18. *Ibid.*, p.207.
19. Toulmin, S., 'Rules and their Relevance for Understanding Human Behavior', in Mischel, T. (ed.), *Understanding Other Persons* (Oxford: Basil Blackwell), 1974, p.199.
20. Hausheer, R., *op.cit.*, 1979, p.xxviii.

Chapter 3

1. This is often referred to as the whig interpretation of history. For a description see for example Carr, E.H., *What is History?* (London: Macmillan), 1961, chapters 1 and 2.
2. Porter, R., *A Social History of Madness* (London: Weidenfeld and Nicolson), 1987, p.39.
3. Dubos, R., *Mirage of Health* (London: George Allen and Unwin Ltd.), 1960, p.112.
4. Porter, R., *op.cit.*, 1987, p.39.
5. Dubos, R., *op.cit.*, 1960, p.112.
6. Jacob, J.M., *Doctors and Rules* (London and New York: Routledge), 1988, p.43.
7. Phillips, E.D., *Greek Medicine* (London: Thames and Hudson), 1973, p.181.
8. Singer, C. and Underwood, E.A., *A Short History of Medicine* 2nd Ed. (Oxford: Clarendon Press), 1962, pp.68-69.
9. Cunningham, A., 'Thomas Sydenham: epidemics, experiment and the 'Good Old Cause'', in French, R. and Wear, A. (eds), *The Medical Revolution in the Seventeenth Century* (Cambridge: Cambridge University Press), 1989, p.189.
10. King, L.S., *Medical Thinking: A Historical Preface* (Princeton: Princeton University Press). 1982, p.271.
11. Singer, C. and Underwood, E.A., *op.cit.*, 1962, p.92.
12. *Ibid.*, p.114.
13. Jewson, N.D., 'The Disappearance of the Sick-Man from Medical Cosmology, 1770-1870' *Sociology* 10:225-244 (1976), p.227.
14. Foucault, M., *The Birth of the Clinic* (London: Tavistock), 1973, p.146 (first published in French, 1963).
15. *Ibid.*, p.146.
16. Jewson, N.D., *op.cit.*, 1976, p.229.

17. Henlé, J., *On Miasmata and Contagie. Translated and with an Introduction by George Rosen* (Baltimore: John Hopkins Press), 1938 (first published in German, 1840).
18. Koch, R., 'Ueber Bakteriologische Forschung' in *Verhandlungen des X. Internationalen Medicinischen Congresses Berlin, 4-9 August 1890* (Berlin: Hirschwald), 1891, pp.35-47.
19. Sattler, E.E., *A History of Tuberculosis from the Time of Sylvius to the Present Day* (Cincinnati: R. Clarke & Co.), 1883, Preface p.V.
20. Dubos, R., *op.cit.*, 1960, p.109.
21. Canguilhem, G., *On the Normal and the Pathological* (Dordrecht: Reidel), 1978, pp.11-12 (originally published in French in 1966).
22. Dubos, R., *op.cit.*, 1960, p.109.
23. Porter, R., *op.cit.*, 1987, p.11.
24. Pagel, W., 'Humoral Pathology. A Lingering Anachronism in the History of Tuberculosis' *Bulletin of the History of Medicine* 29:299-308 (1955), p.300.
25. Webster, C., *From Paracelsus to Newton* (Cambridge: Cambridge University Press), 1982, p.12.
26. Foucault, M., *op.cit.*, 1973, p.146.
27. McKeown, T., *The Role of Medicine* (Oxford: Blackwell), 1979.
28. Armstrong, D., 'The Emancipation of Biographical Medicine' *Social Science and Medicine* 13A:1-8 (1979).

Chapter 4

1. Cochrane, A.L., *Effectiveness and Efficiency* (London: The Nuffield Provincial Hospitals Trust), 1972.
2. McKeown, T., *The Role of Medicine* (Oxford: Blackwell), 1979.
3. Illich, I., *Limits to Medicine* (London: Marion Boyars), 1976.
4. *Ibid.*, pp.270-271.
5. Horrobin, D.F., *Medical Hubris - A Reply to Ivan Illich* (Edinburgh: Churchill Livingstone), 1978, p.81.
6. Fulford, K.W.M., *Moral Theory and Medical Practice* (Cambridge: Cambridge University Press), 1989, Preface p.xiii.
7. Sedgwick, P., *Psycho Politics* (London: Pluto Press), 1982, p.27.
8. Boorse, C., 'On the Distinction Between Disease and Illness' *Philosophy and Public Affairs* 5:49-68 (1975).
9. Fulford, K.W.M., *op.cit.*, 1989, p.263.
10. Dubos, R., *Mirage of Health* (London: George Allen and Unwin Ltd.), 1960, p.218.
11. *Ibid.*, p.219.

12. *Ibid.*, p.219.
13. *Ibid.*, p.218.
14. *Ibid.*, p.219.
15. Cassell, E.J., *The Nature of Suffering and the Goals of Medicine* (Oxford: Oxford University Press), 1991, Preface p.vii.
16. *Ibid.*, p.232.

Chapter 5

1. Ten Have, H.A.M.J., 'Knowledge and Practice in European Medicine: The Case of Infectious Diseases' in Ten Have, H.A.M.J., Kimsma, G.K. and Spicker, S.F. (eds), *The Growth of Medical Knowledge* (Dordrecht: Kluwer Academic Publishers), 1990, p.17.
2. Koch, R., 'Ueber Bakteriologische Forschung' in *Verhandlungen des X. Internationalen Medicinischen Congresses Berlin 4-9 August 1890* (Berlin: Hirschwald), 1891, pp.35-47.
3. Adapted from Wright, P. and Treacher, A. (eds), *The Problem of Medical Knowledge* (Edinburgh, Edinburgh University Press), 1982. and Mishler, E.G., *Social Contexts of Health, Illness and Patient Care* (Cambridge: Cambridge University Press), 1981.
4. Wulff, H.R., 'Function and Value of Medical Knowledge in Modern Diseases.' in Ten Have, H.A.M.J., Kimsma, G.K. and Spicker, S.F. (eds), *The Growth of Medical Knowledge* (Dordrecht: Kluwer Academic Publishers), 1990.
5. Thung, P.J., 'The Growth of Medical Knowledge: An Epistemological Exploration' in Ten Have, H.A.M.J., Kimsma, G.K. and Spicker, S.F. (eds), *The Growth of Medical Knowledge* (Dordrecht: Kluwer Academic Publishers), 1990.
6. Virchow, R., 'One Hundred Years of General Pathology' (originally published in German in 1895) in *Disease, Life and Man* translated by Rather, L.J., (Stanford: Stanford University Press), 1958, p.192.
7. Greaves, D., 'Disease Concepts Models and Classification in Western Medicine - Illustrated by Reference to Pulmonary Tuberculosis and Coronary Heart Disease' *Society for the Social History of Medicine Bulletin* 24:31-35 (1979), p.32.
8. King, L.S., 'What is Disease?' *Philosophy of Science* 21:193-203 (1954), p.200.
9. Payer, L., *Medicine and Culture* (London: Victor Gollancz Ltd.), 1990, pp.86-90.
10. Midgley, M., *Can't We Make Moral Judgements?* (Bristol: The Bristol Press), 1991.

11. Butler, S. *Erewhon* (Trubner and Co.), 1872, chapter 10.
12. Boorse, C., 'On the Distinction between Disease and Illness' *Philosophy and Public Affairs* 5:57-58 (1975).
13. Chang, J., *Wild Swans* (New York: Simon and Schuster), 1991, pp.24-25.
14. Engelhardt, H.T., 'Medical Knowledge and Medical Action: Competing Visions' in Ten Have, H.A.M.J., Kimsma, G.K. and Spicker, S.F. (eds), *The Growth of Medical Knowledge* (Dordrecht: Kluwer Academic Publishers), 1990, p.63.
15. King, L.S., *Medical Thinking: A Historical Preface* (Princeton: Princeton University Press), 1982, pp.11-12.
16. Ludwik Fleck developed his philosophical ideas in the 1920s and 1930s and his best known work is *Genesis and Development of a Scientific Fact* translated by Bradley, F. and Trenn, T.J., (Chicago: University of Chicago Press), 1979 (originally published in German in 1935).
17. Bhaskar, R., *A Realist Theory of Science* 2nd Ed. (Leeds: Leeds Books Ltd.), 1978, p.70.
18. *Ibid.*, p.142.
19. Fleck, L., 'Some Specific Features of the Medical Way of Thinking' (A lecture delivered at the 4th meeting of the Society of Lovers of the History of Medicine at Lwow in 1927). Translated by Cohen, R.S. and Schnelle, T. (eds), in *Cognition and Fact* (Dordrecht: Reidel), 1986, p.44.
20. King, L.S., *op.cit.*, 1982, p.282.
21. *Ibid.*, pp.311-312.

Chapter 6

1. Healy, D., *The Suspended Revolution - Psychiatry and Psychotherapy Re-examined* (London: Faber and Faber), 1990.
2. Kraepelin, E., *Psychiatrica* 4th Ed. (Leipzig), 1893.
3. Described in Hill, D., *The Politics of Schizophrenia* (Lanham: University Press of America), 1983, p.75.
4. Bleuler, E., *Dementia Praecox or the Group of Schizophrenias* translated by Zinkin, J. (New York: International Universities Press), 1950 (first published in German, 1911).
5. Pilowsky, L.S., 'Understanding Schizophrenia' *British Medical Journal* 305:327-328 (1992).
6. Boyle, M., 'The Non-Discovery of Schizophrenia?' in Bentall, R.P. (ed.), *Reconstructing Schizophrenia* (London and New York: Routledge), 1990.
7. Bentall, R.P., 'The Syndromes and Symptoms of Psychosis' in Bentall, R.P. (ed.), *Reconstructing Schizophrenia* (London and New York: Routledge), 1990.

8. Birchwood, M., Hallett, S. and Preston, M., *Schizophrenia* (London: Longman), 1988, p.18.
9. *Ibid.*, p.352.
10. Pilgrim, D., 'Competing Histories of Madness' in Bentall, R.P. (ed.), *Reconstructing Schizophrenia* (London and New York: Routledge), 1990, p.229. The phrase 'insanity is purely a disease of the brain' is a quote from an editorial in the *Journal of Mental Science* of 1858.
11. Goffman, E., *Asylums* (Garden City, New York: Anchor Books), 1961.
12. Scheff, T., *Being Mentally Ill: A Sociological Theory* (London: Weidenfeld and Nicolson), 1966.
13. Szasz, T.S., 'The Myth of Mental Illness' *American Psychologist* 15:113-118 (1960).
14. Laing, R.D., *The Divided Self* (London: Tavistock), 1960.
15. Bentall, R.P., *op.cit.*, p.34.
16. Venables, P.H., 'Longitudinal Research on Schizophrenia' in Bentall, R.P. (ed.), *Reconstructing Schizophrenia* (London and New York: Routledge), 1990.
17. Calman, M., *Preventing Coronary Heart Disease* (London and New York: Routledge), 1991, p.1.
18. Leibowitz, J.O., *The History of Coronary Heart Disease* (London: Wellcome Institute of the History of Medicine), 1970.
19. Marmot, M., 'Facts, Opinions and Affaires Du Coeur' *American Journal of Epidemiology* 103:519-525 (1976).
20. *Ibid.*, p.520.
21. Fleck, L., *Genesis and Development of a Social Fact* translated by Bradley, F. and Trenn, T.J., (Chicago: University of Chicago Press), 1979 (originally published in German in 1935).
22. Wright, P. and Treacher, A. (eds), *The Problem of Medical Knowledge* (Edinburgh: Edinburgh University Press), 1982, p.10.
23. *Ibid.*, p.14.
24. Bloor, M., 'Bishop Berkeley and the Adenotonsillectomy Enigma, an Exploration of Variation in the Social Construction of Medical Disposals' *Sociology* 10:43-61 (1976), pp.58-59.
25. Bartley, M., 'Coronary Heart Disease and the Public Health 1850-1983' *Sociology of Health and Illness* 7:289-313 (1985).
26. *Ibid.*, p.309.
27. *Ibid.*, p.309.
28. Described in Hill, D., *op.cit.*, p.226.
29. For example Murphy, H.B.M., Wittkower, E.D., Fried, J. and Ellenberger, H., 'A Cross-Cultural Survey of Schizophrenic Symptomatology' *International Journal of Social Psychiatry* 9:237-249 (1963).

30. Young, M. and Turnbull, H.M., 'An Analysis of Data Collected by the Status Lymphaticus Investigation Committee' *Journal of Pathology and Bacteriology* 34:213-258 (1931).
31. Susan Sontag explores this theme in relation to tuberculosis and cancer in - Sontag, S., *Illness as Metaphor* (New York: Vintage Books), 1978; and Linnie Price has suggested that CHD lends itself to a similar interpretation in - Price, L., 'Epidemiology, Medical Sociology, and Coronary Heart Disease' *Radical Community Medicine* 15:10-15 (1983).

Chapter 7

1. Parkins, R.A. and Pegrum, G.D., 'Introduction' to *The Basis of Clinical Diagnosis* 2nd Ed. (London: Pitman Medical), 1979.
2. Stimson, G. and Webb, B., *Going to See the Doctor* (London: Routledge and Kegan Paul), 1975, pp.43-44.
3. Cassell, E.J., *The Nature of Suffering and the Goals of Medicine* (Oxford: Oxford University Press), 1991, p.96.
4. Polanyi, M., *Personal Knowledge* (London: Routledge & Kegan Paul), 1958, p.17.
5. Cassell, E.J., *op.cit.*, 1991, pp.230-231.
6. Cassell, E.J., *op.cit.*, 1991, p.232.
7. Cassell, E.J., *op.cit.*, 1991, p.235.
8. Malinowski, B., *Magic, Science, Religion and Other Essays* first published 1925 (New York: Doubleday Anchor Books), 1954, p90.
9. Balint, M., *The Doctor, His Patient and the Illness* 2nd Ed. (London: Pitman Medical), 1964, p.229.
10. *Ibid.*, p.229.
11. Trollope, A., *Doctor Thorne* first published 1858 (Cambridge, Mass.: Riverside Press), 1959, p.127.
12. Balint, E., 'The 'Flash' Technique - Its Freedom and Its Discipline' chapter 2 in Balint, E. and Norell, J.S. (eds), *Six Minutes for the Patient* (London: Tavistock), 1973.
13. This analysis of placebos derives in part from Greaves, D.A., *The Role of Principles in Medical Ethics - Illustrated by Two Examples* (M.A. Dissertation: University of London), 1989.
14. Vogel, A.V., Goodwin, J.S and Goodwin. J.M., 'The Therapeutics of Placebo' *American Family Physician* 22:105-109 (1980).
15. *The Concise Oxford Dictionary* 6th Ed. (Oxford: Oxford University Press). 1976.
16. Bok, S., 'The Ethics of Giving Placebos' *Scientific American* 231:17-23 (1974).

17. Cabot, R.C., *Social Service and the Art of Healing* (New York: Moffat, Yard & Co.), 1909, p.169.
18. Polanyi, M., *op.cit.*, 1958, p.17.
19. Brody, H., *The Healer's Power* (New Haven and London: Yale University Press), 1992, pp.256-257.
20. Berger, J. and Mohr, J., *A Fortunate Man* first published 1967 (Harmondsworth: Penguin), 1969, p.76.
21. *Ibid.*, p.77.
22. Brody, H., *op.cit.*, 1992. This book contains an extended discussion of these opposing forces.
23. Brody, H., *Placebos and the Philosophy of Medicine* (Chicago: University of Chicago Press), 1980, pp.94-95.
24. Appelbaum, P.S., Lidz, C.W. and Meisel, A., *Informed Consent* (New York and Oxford: Oxford University Press), 1987, p.263.
25. King, J., 'Informed Consent' *IME Bulletin* Supplement No.3 (Dec 1986).
26. Carnerie, F., 'Crisis and Informed Consent: Analysis of a Law-Medicine Malocclusion' *American Journal of Law and Medicine* 12:55-97 (1987), p.55.
27. Merskey, H., 'An Ethical Issue in the Psychotherapy of Pain and Other Symptoms' *Bioethics* 4:22-32 (1990).
28. *Ibid.*, p.32.
29. Harris, L. and Associates, 'Views of Informed Consent and Decisionmaking: Parallel Surveys of Physicians and the Public' in The President's Commission Report *Making Health Care Decisions: Appendices* (Washington, D.C.: U.S. Government Printing Office), 1982.
30. The President's Commission Report, *Making Health Care Decisions: Appendices* (Washington, D.C.: U.S. Government Printing Office), 1982. p.402.
31. *Ibid.*, p.403.
32. Jacob, J.M., *Doctors and Rules* (London: Routledge) 1988, p.170.

Chapter 8

1. Wulff, H., 'Alternative Medicine' pp.174-178 in *Rational Klinik* 3rd Ed. (Copenhagen: Uunksgaard), 1987.
2. Sullivan, M.D., 'Placebo Controls and Epistemic Control in Orthodox Medicine' *Journal of Medicine and Philosophy* 18:213-231 (1993), p.218.
3. Maxwell, R.J., Editorial 'The Osteopaths Bill' *British Medical Journal* 306:1556-1557 (1993).
4. Maclean, U., *Magical Medicine* (Harmondsworth: Penguin Press), 1971, p.143.

5. Baron, R.J., 'An Introduction to Medical Phenomenology: I Can't Hear You While I'm Listening' *Annals of Internal Medicine* 103:606-611 (1985), p.607.

6. Horobin, G., 'Professional Mystery: the Maintenance of Charisma in General Medical Practice' in Dingwall, R. and Lewis, P. (eds), *The Sociology of the Professions: Lawyers, Doctors and Others* (London: Macmillan), 1983.

7. For an account of the development of homeopathy see for example - Danciger, E., *The Emergence of Homeopathy* (London: Century Hutchinson), 1987.

8. Adapted from Bayley, C., 'Homeopathy' *Journal of Medicine and Philosophy* 18:129-145 (1993).

9. Kleijnen, J., Knipschild, P. and ter Riet, G., 'Clinical Trials in Homeopathy,' *British Medical Journal* 302:316-323 (1991). This review of clinical trials provides the most comprehensive assessment to date.

10. Sullivan, M.D. *op.cit.*, 1993, p.229.

Chapter 9

1. Jonas, H., *The Imperative of Responsibility* (Chicago and London: University of Chicago Press), 1984, p.9.

2. Reiser, S.J., *Medicine and the Reign of Technology* (Cambridge,: Cambridge University Press), 1978, p.171.

3. *Ibid.*, p.228.

4. Cochrane, A.L., *Effectiveness and Efficiency* (The Nuffield Provincial Hospitals Trust), 1972.

5. Pope, C. and Mays, N., 'Opening the Black Box: an Encounter in the Corridors of Health Services Research' *British Medical Journal* 306:315-318 (1993).

6. Chalmers, A.F., 'Epidemiology and the Scientific Method' *International Journal of Health Services* 12:659-666 (1982), p.661.

7. *Ibid.*, p.662.

8. See for example Kennedy, I., 'The Law and Ethics of Informed Consent and Randomised Controlled Trials' in Kennedy, I., *Treat Me Right* (Oxford: Clarendon Press), 1988.

9. Chalmers, A.F., *Science and Its Fabrication* (Milton Keynes: Open University Press), 1990, p.6.

10. Congressional Office of Technology Assessment *Assessing the Efficacy and Safety of Medical Technologies* (Washington D.C.), 1978.

11. Stocking, B., 'Factors Influencing the Effectiveness of Mechanisms to Control Medical Technology' in Stocking, B. (ed.), *Expensive Health Technologies* (Oxford: Oxford University Press), 1988, p.24.

12. Jennett, B., *High Technology Medicine* (Oxford: Oxford University Press), 1986.
13. Cassell, E.J., *The Nature of Suffering* (Oxford: Oxford University Press), 1991, pp.44-45.
14. Swales, J.D., et al. 'Treating Mild Hypertension. Report of the British Hypertension Working Party' *British Medical Journal* 298:694-698 (1989).
15. Dollery, C., *The End of an Age of Optimism* (The Nuffield Provincial Hospitals Trust), 1978.

Chapter 10

1. Beveridge Report *Social Insurance and Allied Services* (London: HMSO), 1942, p.105 para. 270(3).
2. In 1952, for example, the government set up the Guillebaud Committee to examine this issue. *Committee of Enquiry into the Cost of the National Health Service* (London: HMSO), 1956.
3. Greaves, D., 'The Ethics of the Internal Market' in Szawarski, Z. and Evans, D. (eds), *Solidarity, Justice and Health Care Priorities* (Linköping: Linköping Collaborating Centre), 1993, pp.77-87.
4. Evans, M., 'The "Management" of Demand for Health Care' *International Journal of Health Care Quality Assurance* 3, No. 2:5-10 (1990), p.5.
5. Payer, L., *Medicine and Culture* (London: Gollancz), 1990, p.101.
6. Scheff, T.J., 'Decision Rules, Types of Error, and their Consequences in Medical Diagnosis' *Behavioral Science* 8:97-107 (1963), p.97.
7. Cassell, E.J., 'Error in Medicine' in Engelhardt Jr., H.T. and Callahan, D. (eds), *Knowledge Value and Belief* (New York: The Hastings Center), 1977, p.303.
8. *Ibid.*, p.304.
9. Ten Have, H., 'Physicians' Priorities - Patients' Expectations' in Szawarski, Z. and Evans, D. (eds), *Solidarity Justice and Health Care Priorities* (Linköping: Linköping Collaborating Centre), 1993, pp.42-52.
10. Callahan, D., 'Pursuing a Peaceful Death' *Hastings Center Report* 23, No. 4:33-38 (1993).

Chapter 11

1. Van der Post, L., *Jung and the Story of Our Time* (London: The Hogarth Press), 1976, pp.62-63.

2. Wisdom, J., *Paradox and Discovery* (Oxford: Basil Blackwell), 1965, pp.137-138.

3. Horobin, G., 'Professional Mystery: the Maintenance of Charisma in General Medical Practice' in Dingwall, R. and Lewis, P. (eds), *The Sociology of the Professions: Lawyers, Doctors and Others* (London: Macmillan), 1983, p.94.

4. Wartofsky, M.W., Editorial, *Journal of Medicine and Philosophy* 3:265-272 (1978), p.267.

5. Toulmin, S., 'Knowledge and Art in the Practice of Medicine: Clinical Judgment and Historical Reconstruction' in Delkeskamp-Hayes, C. and Cutter, M.A.G. (eds), *Science, Technology and the Art of Medicine* (Dordrecht: Kluwer Academic Publishers), 1993, p.247.

6. Brody, H., *The Healer's Power* (New Haven and London: Yale University Press), 1992, p.263.

7. Cassell, E.J., 'Making and Escaping Moral Decisions' *Hastings Center Studies* 53-62 (1973), p.62.

8. Ladd, J., 'Physicians and Society: Tribulations of Power and Responsibility' in Spicker, S.F., Healey, J.M. and Engelhardt, H.T. (eds), *The Law-Medicine Relation: A Philosophical Exploration* (Dordrecht: Reidel), 1981, p.44.

9. Gellner, E., 'The Savage and the Modern Mind' in Horton, R. and Finnegan, R. (eds), *Modes of Thought* (London: Faber and Faber), 1973, p.180.

10. Midgley, M., *Science as Salvation* (London and New York: Routledge), 1992, pp.223-224.

11. Callahan, D., *Setting Limits* (New York: Simon and Schuster), 1987, p.60.

Bibliography

Bennet, G., *The Wound and the Doctor* (London: Secker and Warburg), 1987.

Berger, J. and Mohr, J., *A Fortunate Man* (London: Allen Lane, The Penguin Press), 1967.

Brody, H., *The Healer's Power* (New Haven and London: Yale University Press), 1992.

Canguilhem, G., *On the Normal and the Pathological* (Dordrecht: Reidel), 1978. (originally published in French in 1966).

Cassell, E.J., *The Nature of Suffering and the Goals of Medicine* (Oxford: Oxford University Press), 1991.

Cochrane, A.L., *Effectiveness and Efficiency* (London: The Nuffield Provincial Hospital Trust), 1972.

Delkeskamp-Hayes, C. and Cutter, M.A.G. (eds), *Science Technology and the Art of Medicine* (Dordrecht: Kluwer Academic Publishers), 1993.

Dubos, R., *Mirage of Health* (London: George Allen and Unwin Ltd.), 1960.

Fleck, L., *Genesis and Development of a Scientific Fact* translated by Bradley, F. and Trenn, T.J., (Chicago: University of Chicago Press), 1979 (originally published in German in 1935).

Fulford, K.W.M., *Moral Theory and Medical Practice* (Cambridge: Cambridge University Press), 1989.

Illich, I., *Limits to Medicine* (London: Marion Boyars), 1976.

Jacob, J.M., *Doctors and Rules* (London and New York: Routledge), 1988.

Kennedy, I., *The Unmasking of Medicine* (London: George Allen and Unwin Ltd.), 1981.

King, L.S., *Medical Thinking: A Historical Preface* (Princeton: Princeton University Press), 1982.

McKeown, T., *The Role of Medicine* (Oxford: Blackwell), 1979.

Payer, L., *Medicine and Culture* (London: Victor Gollancz Ltd.), 1990.

Reiser, S.J., *Medicine and the Reign of Technology* (Cambridge: Cambridge University Press), 1978.

Shorter, E., *Bedside Manners* (New York: Simon and Schuster), 1985.

Ten Have, H.A.M.J., Kinsma, G.K. and Spicker, S.F. (eds), *The Growth of Medical Knowledge* (Dordrecht: Kluwer Academic Publishers), 1990.

Index